Praise for *True Strength*

"This actor has a real and really interesting story to tell . . . This is the story of a man who had taken from him that which made up the entirety of his persona: strength. And how he recovered." —*Asbury Park Press*

"Sorbo is candid about the hopelessness and resentment that characterized his slow recovery, his frustration with contradictory medical advice and holistic therapies of varying effectiveness and the stress his condition placed on his new marriage." —*Kirkus Reviews*

"[A] compelling memoir . . . Throughout his chatty tale, he drops enough Hollywood names to make any *Us Weekly* reader happy." —*Booklist*

"A story of inspiration and hope through the most trying of situations. It should be read by everyone so that they can understand, even if just a little bit, how it feels to live through a stroke or other life altering medical issue, and come out on the other side spiritually renewed." —ThirdOptionMen.org

"A gripping account of Sorbo's illness and gradual recovery."
—*Huffington Post*

"As much an inspirational story as a narrative about the former model's rise to cable stardom, the often surprisingly candid memoir offers a look at the effects long-term debilitation can have on relationships and careers . . . A compelling look at a life temporarily derailed." —A.V. Club (*The Onion*)

"His story is no mythic journey; it's all too human, and well worth reading." —Shelf Awareness for Readers

"*True Strength* has a deliberately upbeat tone and message, with Sorbo working his way back into acting and becoming head of a mentoring program for inner-city teens. This is all very admirable and will be inspirational . . . Certainly his story is worth cheering." —InfoDad.com

"*True Strength* covers the stunning transformation of how a powerful man found himself brought low, and how embracing his frailties saved him from missing out on what really matters: love and family . . . The narrative voice is genuine and powerful, with Sorbo's infectious positive attitude and guileless approach to success." —*San Francisco Book Review*

TRUE STRENGTH

MY JOURNEY FROM HERCULES TO MERE MORTAL
AND HOW NEARLY DYING SAVED MY LIFE

KEVIN SORBO

Da Capo Press

A Member of the Perseus Books Group

This book is the creation of research and memory. Some of the names of people in this book have been changed to protect their privacy.

In no way is this book intended to replace, countermand, or conflict with the advice given to you by your own physician. The ultimate decision concerning care should be made between you and your doctor. We strongly recommend you follow his or her advice. Information in this book is general and is offered with no guarantees on the part of the authors or Da Capo Press. The authors and publisher disclaim all liability in connection with the use of this book.

Editorial production by *Marra*thon Production Services. www.marrathon.net

DESIGN BY JANE RAESE
Text set in Utopia

Library of Congress Cataloging-in-Publication Data is available for this book.

ISBN 978-0-306-82036-6 (hardcover)
ISBN 978-0-7382-1602-7 (paperback)
ISBN 978-0-306-82055-7 (e-book)

Published by Da Capo Press
A Member of the Perseus Books Group
www.dacapopress.com

Da Capo Press books are available at special discounts for bulk purchases in the U.S. by corporations, institutions, and other organizations. For more information, please contact the Special Markets Department at the Perseus Books Group, 2300 Chestnut Street, Suite 200, Philadelphia, PA, 19103, or call (800) 810-4145, ext. 5000, or e-mail special.markets@perseusbooks.com.

FIRST DA CAPO PRESS EDITION 2011
FIRST DA CAPO PRESS PAPERBACK EDITION 2012

10 9 8 7 6 5 4 3 2 1

WITH THANKS TO GOD.

FOR MY WIFE, SAM,
who helped me find the words to write this book.

CONTENTS

ACKNOWLEDGMENTS

LIFE IS A CONTACT SPORT, requiring teamwork for a successful game. Similarly, this book would not exist without the efforts of a dedicated lineup, for which I am eternally grateful. They are, in no particular order:

Robert Frost, for the discernment to choose the playing field that wanted wear.

Ardis and Lynn Sorbo (Mom and Dad), for the coin toss.

All of my doctors, especially but not limited to Dr. Robert Huizenga and Dr. Franklin Moser, without whom I would have had to forfeit the game.

The crew, cast, and producers of *Hercules,* especially Rob Tapert, Eric Greundemann, John Mahaffie, George Lyle, Michael Hurst, and Bruce Campbell for being my tireless teammates, allowing me to selfishly rely on them to carry the ball when I was too weak to go it alone.

Dr. Philip Stutz, Dr. Tony Norie, Steve Rosenbaum and Lee Goral, who gave me a new playbook and helped me improve my game.

Jennifer Gates and Todd Shuster, for being our cheerleaders (mine and the book's.)

Katie McHugh, Jonathan Sainsbury, and Lissa Warren, for their coaching.

Donna Ruthe, for her insights and analysis.

My wife, Sam Sorbo, for keeping my head in the game.

And lastly (but by no means least), my kids, Braeden, Shane and Tavia, for the tackle practice, popcorn, and everything else.

INTRODUCTION

SUDDENLY I WAS AWAKE.

"Don't move."

The words seemed to come from inside my head, low and emphatic.

What was that incessant, droning sound? I was falling backward, but I was not moving.

"Don't move."

I flexed my toes, balled my fists, and counted the tubes in my arms and in my groin, remembering the strict instructions not to reposition myself no matter what, because I might bleed out. That's right . . . bleed out.

It was coming back quickly now. I had blood thinners coursing through my arteries. Something in my arm, no, shoulder, had sent several hundred blood clots down my arm. When they reached an artery too small to pass, they stuck there, blocking any fresh blood and suffocating my flesh. My fingers had slowly turned blue—cold and tingly.

We were attacking back. Heparin, the clot-busting, blood-thinning wonder drug would set everything straight again—I hoped. My arm throbbed—probably the drug's healing effects. I flexed and folded the fingers on my left hand again, lifting it a few inches off the bed to get a look at it. My fingers still felt swollen, but at least they didn't look as blue. I turned my hand and it started to tingle.

I put it down carefully. I did not want to "bleed out." Just like in *Ghostbusters*, I knew "It would be *bad*."

Something was stabbing between my eyes and pooling behind my head—an excruciatingly bright heat. That ceaseless noise wasn't helping at all.

I glanced around me as best as I could without moving my head too much. Yep, I was still in the ICU, with my new friends, a collection of medical machines, ticking away, hanging over the bed to scrutinize my every heartbeat.

But just as I focused on the IV, the heart monitor next to it *disappeared*. What?

I looked carefully, trying to see the monitor in my periphery. No luck. So I refixed my gaze on the heart monitor directly. There it was, doing its job—I presumed.

Apparently, my new blind spot was with me for the long haul. Shit.

I closed my eyes and felt . . . worse. Lightning strikes flashed through the darkness. How was that even possible? Then the dizziness hit, and every small movement generated a new, awful sensation. I was falling, spinning, freezing, floating. Nausea rolled on my tongue like a ball bearing.

That's right: "Don't move."

The bed was a dingy in rough seas. *Oh, no!* I realized, *I'm not supposed to move. How am I going to throw up?*

That's when it hit me how hungry I was. How many days had it been? At least three. I heard the ICU nurses in the hallway, talking, joking, laughing. One of them yelled to the other one, who must've been walking away, "Yeah, that's what *she* said!"

Huh. Is there nothing original anymore, ever?

"Don't move."

Oh, Lord, how I wanted to get up and just walk out of there. My ass was killing me. My back ached, even the skin on it was tender, and my legs were angry for lack of use. I could just feel my muscles slipping off my bones. For the athlete in me, this was torture, but the doctors assured me that this treatment was the only way to save my arm, and even that was still uncertain.

What would I do without my left arm?

Luckily, right then came another wave of nausea to distract me from my speculations. How can a person feel like puking when there is nothing in there? I flexed my feet to give my legs a small release. Boy, that got me even dizzier.

I was on a Tilt-A-Whirl, but there was nothing amusing about it. I just wanted some peace and quiet, to go back to sleep. I wished, for the thousandth time, that the nurses would shut off that infernal generator. Its relentless humming was driving me crazy.

And that's when it finally dawned on me: The sound was coming from *inside* my head. It was that smoldering, wet heat at the base of my skull. Intrinsically, I knew that this was the real problem.

And all the rest of this, the tube in my groin—the one crossing through my heart to deliver the clot-busting medicine directly to my shoulder and arm, the reason I was not permitted to move—was simply a distraction. It was an effective diversion, for now. *Look at that tube.* I pondered with incredulity the precious plastic passing innocuously through my heart, even as my heart kept beating. But the impartial tube, the faithful heart, the treacherous shoulder, the angry throbbing arm, the tingling hand and blue fingers, even my deceitful eyes—none of those sinister concerns could compete with what was happening in my head. My brain was the *thing*.

I understood. Although the end had not yet come, I was teetering on the brink of complete destruction. So I clung clumsily to the distractions of my circumstances in the ICU of this famous hospital. And while I examined this new life, the old one flashed in my memory: playing football in the snow in our front yard with my neighbors, driving alone for the first time in my '67 Ford Mustang, riding the subways in Paris. It all seemed so surreal and fast. Fear is an extraordinary artist, stimulating the mind to reminisce, as if to divine where fairytale meets horror novel.

Through it all I couldn't help but think: What did I do to deserve this?

PART I
DEMIGOD

MINNESOTA BOY

Years ago—not long after I'd first moved to Hollywood—my good friend Tony "The Head" Federico arranged for us to play golf with Joe Pesci. I was a nobody actor and was thrilled. Plus I was (and still am) a golf nut.

So it is Tony (Italian), my buddy Rafe Battiste (Italian), and Joe (yep, Italian), and me. We meet and greet on the first tee, hit our shots, and start walking down the fairway together. Joe is not quite average height—I have close to ten inches on him—but he has an intimidating manner and a strong, irresistible confidence about who he is.

I am walking next to him. Joe squints up at me, and with his clipped, heavy New Jersey drawl (sounding much like the characters he plays), demands, "Sorbo? What the fuck is Sorbo?"

I look at him and say, "I'm Norwegian. One hundred percent."

Without missing a beat he scoffs, "Fuck that! Norwegian! Your name ends with a fucking vowel! You're a fucking Italian!"

We've been friends ever since.

⌒

I'm just your average guy who was blessed with a solid upbringing from good, loving, first-generation Norwegian parents with full American values. I was the fourth of five kids, all boys save for one girl, who was stuck

7

in the middle. We lived on a quiet cul-de-sac (we called it a dead end back in those days) across the street from my best friends, Mark and Dan, whom I still see at least once a year.

Our house had three bedrooms and a bathroom—trust me, nothing fancy on my father's salary as a junior high school teacher. We had a great yard that was surrounded by other sprawling yards with homes similar to mine. Between them, they housed an army of kids and provided a wonderful, magical world to grow up in. At the bottom of our street there was a park with a moat-like street called Clover Circle guarding it. It was perfect for a gaggle of kids to play baseball, football, and basketball as well as to use as a make-out spot when we hit our teen years (yes, Mom and Dad, this did transpire on more than one occasion). Farther down there was Dutch lake, where I would immerse myself in the cold water during the humid Minnesota summers. I'd play on Carlson's raft until the water got too cold in those gusty autumns that heralded another Midwest winter.

The years passed slowly and happily. I don't have the horror stories of childhood that so many seem to remember. I had great parents, a cozy neighborhood, and an unpretentious small town to grow up in, with dedicated coaches and teachers who were instrumental in forming the man I would become.

I was an A-B student throughout my school years, and although I was a jock, I got along with everyone, from the burnouts to the nerds. I loved sports most and entertained dreams of being a professional basketball player. (What jock doesn't?)

When I was eleven my elementary school teachers took our class downtown to the Guthrie Theater in Minneapolis to see *The Merchant of Venice*. A field trip to the city was an exciting reprieve from schoolwork, but this one was more than that—it was the day I fell in love with the stage. Shakespeare convinced me on that afternoon of my love for theater, performance, and language. The actors and how they commanded the attention of everyone in the room mesmerized me. It wasn't "real," and yet they still made people listen, think, laugh, and cry. That was tremendous power. The match had been lit and my passion ignited. Later on, though, I had no idea what to do with that enthusiasm because my parents would never condone a career in Hollywood. And I loved my sports too much to confess my interest in drama to my teammates: They would have crucified me! So I shoved acting onto a back burner. I kept the heat low but always watched the stove.

I enrolled at Moorhead State University in northern Minnesota across the Red River from Fargo, North Dakota. I did continue to play sports, but looking around the field at the other very talented athletes in my Division III university, I soon realized that I needed more realistic plans than to be a football or basketball star. I settled on pursuing a business degree and disclosed to no one my fantasy of making it in Hollywood.

After Christmas break my junior year, I was driving back to Moorhead State on I-94 North in a breezy old Ford Mustang Grande when a Minnesota blizzard struck. My car was quickly engulfed—it was a complete whiteout. I drove slowly, hoping to find an exit with some shelter, like a gas station or restaurant, but that turned out to be pointless on this desolate stretch of highway. (This was well before cell phones.)

There I was, a lone vehicle on the barren frozen tundra, thirty miles south of Fargo/Moorhead. It might as well have been three hundred. Armed with a Snickers bar and a quarter tank of gas—while freezing my ass off—I passionately announced out loud how much I hated the cold. For the umpteenth time. I pounded the steering wheel and shivered.

The shadows of dusk crept in. A snowplow or rescue team might not come until morning. That suspicion was confirmed when the radio blurted that all traffic had been cleared of the stretch of road I was traveling. "Wait!! I'm still stuck out here in this crap!"

I carefully forged ahead through the storm at a blistering five miles per hour, just hoping I would stay on the road. Then . . . THUD!

I hit something. Actually, I had nudged up against something solid—another car. I couldn't go any further, so I got out of my car in the seventy-five-degrees-below-zero-with-wind-chill weather and felt my way over to the car I had bumped into.

I discovered four girls from Concordia College, a private college just blocks from my own. First, I made sure they were all right. Then I took in the new development. Four coeds! Suddenly my prospects didn't seem so dismal.

They informed me that there were two more cars right in front of them and we were all sitting in front of a bridge that was closed off by the now twelve-foot snowdrift. There would be no more driving tonight, that much was clear.

I stayed in my car until it ran out of gas. Then I joined the coeds in their car for warmth. We all still froze, but at least we wouldn't die alone.

I joke now about the coeds, but truth be told, it was a frightening situation. Throughout the night, the talk turned to what-ifs: What if we're not found in time? And we kept our fears stoked with memories of the annual news reports of people freezing to death in similar situations. I tried to concentrate on the other stories—the ones with the happy endings.

It turned out we would be the latter. After a four-hour drive and six hours stalled in the blizzard, a blast of light hit us from behind. One of the cars in front of us had been able to reach the police on their CB radio and tell the rescue squad where we were.

I almost lost two of my toes to frostbite. I had been cold and hungry, contemplating death and thinking about life. That is often the stuff of epiphanies, and there it was: I knew what I wanted to do with my life.

I was no longer content to sit out in the cold. With only one quarter to finish up on my double major in marketing and advertising, I dropped out of school, determined to market and advertise *myself*—and make my life as an actor.

COLD FEET

THE WHOLE IDEA of moving to Los Angeles still intimidated this small-town boy. I knew not a soul out there, so I decided instead to follow Candace, my girlfriend, to Dallas, Texas, where she assured me all kinds of modeling work awaited. She had been modeling around the world for years. There in Dallas I started diving into acting classes and auditioning for commercials.

After eighteen months Candace convinced me to travel to Italy with her. (I didn't need much convincing, by the way.) We spent eight months in Milan, went to Paris for six, then on to Zurich, Hamburg, London, Scandinavia, and Belguim, ending eventually in Munich.

Modeling is the most amazing work if you can get it, and I was lucky enough to get it. My bookings took me to the Canary Islands, Tunisia, and the pyramids in Egypt, where a camel spit at me. Modeling jobs lasted anywhere from a day to two weeks long, and the people hiring wanted to be able to enjoy their work. This training ground was where I first learned that it isn't only about looks or talent; it's equally important to have a personality that others enjoy, or they will find someone else—someone they like better—for the job.

It was an amazing and valuable experience to spend three and a half years in that environment, but eventually I got tired of modeling. I loved the travel it offered, but my creative side was ready to bust out. Candace was tiring of the model life as well. She proposed we move back home to

Minneapolis to get married. She wanted me to take a job working for her stepfather's real estate company. She had big plans for us.

My plans were big too, but that is where the similarities stopped. She didn't believe in my dream to be an actor. Her parents didn't either. Hell, I am sure most people didn't. What was I thinking, after all? That I could just march into Hollywood and announce, "Hey, here I am!"? The easy money is on disappointment: Most people fail in show business. Even with small successes, the chances of making a career of acting are close to nil.

Stupid or smart, I believed in me. Candace's insistence on her own dream forced my hand. I committed, instead, to move to Hollywood and prove myself.

"I can't believe you're walking out on us!"

"I can't believe you won't let me live my dream," I answered. Ah, the drama of youth!

I rode the midnight train to Milan for one last visit. After all, this was where my European journey started; it seemed only right that this was where it should end. I stayed up all night, leaning out an open window of the train as it lumbered through the small, sleeping towns of the Bavarian Alps. The purple, star-filled sky and warm breezes prompted me to replay the previous five years of my life. My three-month European summer vacation had ended up being three years of "the road less traveled," putting my plans for what I felt was my destiny on hold.

There are no regrets, though. I had grown up over there—matured.

A sweet sadness came over me, but it felt good. The heavy shell cracked and light shone in, daring me to come out. I was filled with anticipation.

After three final months in Milan I headed home for another family Christmas in Mound, Minnesota—and a big life shift.

~

In June 1986 I landed in Los Angeles, working in commercials to support myself: Doritos on the beach, Pert shampoo at the gym. I shot a Japanese chewing gum commercial and had to smoke for it (disgusting) and a hilarious one for beer as an Indiana Jones–type discovering a genie in a lantern: "It says '*Bud* Lite,' not '*rub* light'!" It was a step in the right direction, and I loved it: being on set and watching the crew, the directors, and producers. Any time in front of the camera was good for me, just to put those miles on.

The commercial world is very competitive. I worked my tail off and made my luck happen. Nothing was handed to me. No uncle in the business. I dedicated myself and took the wisdom of a friend in Minnesota who reminded me that it's called show *business*, not show *show*.

My apartment in Santa Monica was a third-floor walk-up unit. Nothing fancy, but I didn't need fancy. I needed functional, and it was a short walk to the beach and a five-minute bike ride to Gold's Gym, which soon became my second home.

Gold's Gym was *the* workout palace for bodybuilders and power lifters, and even for the rest of us guys who just needed a good, serious workout. It was not, by any standards, a social club. In a warehouse building, blocks from the beach, it was big but not spacious, and it reeked of brute strength, blood, sweat, and steroids. This was where I went to pound out the frustrations of my day. This was where I bench-pressed away the traffic, the lazy casting directors, the rude assistants, the snobby actor-types, and, most importantly, the unavoidable, ubiquitous rejection.

After the gym I would often take a lengthy bike ride or rollerblade along the miles of pristine beachfront that the Los Angeles seaboard offers. From Pacific Palisades to Hermosa, Manhattan, or Redondo Beach, the spectacular ocean, with its cool, cleansing breezes, provided another type of respite from the pressures of my insatiable drive for success.

Newton stated that a body in motion tends to remain in motion unless acted upon by an external force. That was me. I didn't work out to stay in shape; I was in great shape because I craved exercise. Physical exertion was my coping mechanism for a high-stress career. While I worked out on the Stairmaster, I read scripts or studied lines. If I had downtime, I wouldn't sit on the couch; I'd be on the move. When I had a headache, I'd go for a jog on the beach. My buddies from home started calling their visits "Boot Camp Sorbo" for the grueling workouts I subjected them to, complaining they needed a vacation from their vacation!

After I had been in LA for a few years my hard work was paying off. I was booking so many jobs that my commercial reputation began to catch up to me. I would show up at an audition and the guys, most of whom I knew by then, would say, "Okay, might as well go home, guys. Sorbs is here, now!" If the commercial shot out of the country, I inevitably got it. Don't ask me why; it just happened. In the three years leading up to *Hercules* I shot forty commercials. I knew I was doing well when my commercial agent showed me on the casting notice that the client was looking for a "Kevin Sorbo" type. Of course, I did not get that job.

MR. WRONG

I WAS WORKING STEADILY in commercials and also landing regular TV guest roles. The demanding acting classes I enjoyed were paying off. Life was good, I guess, except for my love life. I was a driven man; I didn't have time to fall in love.

Don't get me wrong—I was looking. But the exploring and experimenting was starting to bore me. I just couldn't find the right girl. I had dated this one girl for three years—a great woman—but I just couldn't give her what she wanted. Yeah, typical male excuse, I know: "It's me, not you." But it was true. It was, in fact, me. I wasn't ready for marriage, and I hurt her when I walked away. I know because for a long time she really disliked me, to put it politely. My buddies back in Minnesota gave me a hard time for that one too. "Boobs and bucks! What are you, an idiot?" She came from big money, but I am not the type to marry someone for financial security. I preferred to make it on my own.

I remember meeting a gorgeous, leggy blond at a big party that my modeling agent, Nina Blanchard, threw back in 1986 to welcome new models to Los Angeles. I had just moved to Los Angeles. Jennifer was statuesque and stunning as she stood in the entry with Nina. I was not without my own charms, though, so I walked up to them both, proffering glasses of white wine, and Nina offered a gracious introduction.

Jennifer and I immediately hit it off. We both definitely felt the chemistry as we talked and joked the night away, managing to ensure that we sat next to each other at the dinner table. We got caught up in our conversation, and after dinner finished we moved to an intimate corner by the pool behind the house, where she immediately lit up a cigarette.

The cozy property overlooked the sparkling lights of West Hollywood. It was glamorous and romantic and seductive, but after about an hour outside—and three or four cigarettes—I made the excuse that it was late, and I prepared to go. She looked me over, a puzzled expression on her face.

I offered a sad smile. "You're probably wondering why I'm not asking you for your number."

She candidly admitted she was. Boy, she was beautiful. This was such a waste.

"I can't date you," I gently explained. "You smoke."

She did a slow burn right in front of my eyes. Clearly, she was not accustomed to being rejected. "Wow. Um, wow. You would let something that trivial get in the way of a relationship?"

I cut to the chase. "Yeah, pretty much. It's just not that trivial to me, I guess. Sorry," I shrugged.

"Fuck off," she said, pushing past me back into the house.

What can I say? I was picky. I had kissed smokers before and knew it was an incredible turnoff for me. But I deserved that; I had wasted her time, and Hollywood is not the place where a girl can afford to waste even one evening.

I met another woman, Tiffany, at a commercial audition. We struck up a flirty conversation during the long wait, and sparks flew between us. That Friday I took Tiffany to dinner at an upscale, trendy Italian restaurant where the "who" of the "who's who" hung out. She picked it, knowing the city far better than I did.

Tiffany was wearing skin-tight jeans and a blousy white top, and beneath the makeup and feathered hair was an eager girl, desperate to get ahead in the industry. I've always admired drive and determination; I identify with it, which may be why I was attracted to her in the first place. Well, that, and she was hot too.

When we entered said hot spot she called the maître d' by name and they kissed on both cheeks. Very European, I thought. On the way to our table Tiffany spotted some friends who were eating and stopped briefly to chat. The food and smells were tantalizing, and I was hungry and slightly impatient as she flitted to yet another table to talk. I also found it odd that she did not introduce me at either table.

It was a busy night and the place was hopping. Finally, we sat down at a cozy table by the windows. I was looking forward to getting to know my companion a little better. "How long have you been in LA?" I asked her. "Oh, four years, but it feels like forever. How about you?" I never got the chance to answer. Tiffany glanced up over her menu and waved to another group of people she obviously knew. "Excuse me. I will be right back." They were just leaving, so she ran over to kiss and hug them goodbye. I was starting to get a bit miffed with the disappearing act, but I decided patience was called for. This was, after all, Hollywood, and connections and who you know can be the key to your big break.

When the waiter brought our drinks, she ran back over to ask for a dinner salad and shrimp pasta, and I ordered a *prosciutto e melone* and steak. Then off she went to talk to a fourth group of friends. *Seriously?* She motioned in my direction, pointing me out to her friends. I smiled and waved good-naturedly. Then I watched, mystified, as she moved over to yet another table. As they served our starters, she came back to her seat and we began to eat.

"You sure know a lot of people," I offered.

"Yeah. I make friends a lot. Oh my god! See that table that is just sitting down over there?" She pointed, they saw her, then she waved excitedly. "I met the girl at Helena's last week. That is so strange to run into her here. Plus I'm pretty sure that's a guy I dated a couple of times last year. I have to go say hi. I'll be right back . . ."

I ate alone for a few minutes as my patience ran out. Clearly I was the only one on this date. I stewed for a bit longer and then flagged down a waiter.

"I'd like to order us a bottle of Dom Perignon, please."

Now, I knew this was no cheap bottle of champagne, and sure enough, it got her undivided attention when she returned to our table. She was very impressed, apologizing for all the "distractions."

We toasted the evening, new beginnings, and some other nonsense, and then I announced that I needed the restroom. I joked that it was my turn to leave her at the table. Fake laughter ensued.

"Okay, I'll meet you back here, then, in a few!" she said as I walked away. She stood up, too, to find more friends.

I calmly went toward the bathroom but cut through the kitchen, getting surprised looks from the chef and his staff. I tipped the valet guy and never looked back, though I did regret leaving behind that steak.

Yeah, being a gentleman with a Midwest upbringing, I had felt compelled to leave a few C-notes under my plate to cover the bill.

But I kind of hope she didn't find them.

One day late in 1991 I was chatting with a few of my fellow actors in Richard Brander's acting class. A friend overheard me mention that I was looking for a new manager and told me he had a great one. He passed on the info to me and I set up a meeting with her.

Enter Beverlee Dean.

I drove over to her Beverly Hills apartment where she lived and worked. The ground-floor apartments were actually below ground, with windows at street level. I always felt odd walking past people having dinner or watching TV, with them looking up at my feet.

Beverlee buzzed me in through the wrought-iron security gate to the pink, four-level 1950s building, and I walked up a half-flight of stairs to her door. She called out to me, "Let yourself in!"

The living room was cozy with old-fashioned furniture. I saw Beverlee, a diminutive woman in her mid-fifties, seated on a floral couch, surrounded by papers and scripts.

"Oh my God!"

Beverlee had puffy, bleached hair and an animated face. Her very keen eyes were wrapped in oversized black glasses, and those eyes were trained intently on me. "Oh my God!" She jumped up to stand, giving her only marginally more height. Papers fluttered. "Come *over* here!" she exclaimed. "Oh my God! What is wrong with you? Do you do drugs?"

She wore black leggings and, on her large torso, a black-and rust-patterned shiny shirt that fell to her knees. She gave the impression of one of those wooden dolls with legs suspended under an umbrella dress—if you start them walking downhill, they self-propel.

"No! God, no. I . . ."

"Are you high? Where have you been?"

"Uh, I'm not sure what you mean. Our appointment was for two o'-clock, and it's just two now. Sorry if—"

"No, no, no. That's not what I mean. I mean, what's *wrong* with you?" she barked. "Have you been hiding under a rock? What have you been *doing* all this time? Why aren't you a star? You should be a *star.*"

"Oh. Well, uh, thank you, I guess." It sounded like more of an accusation than a compliment.

"Let me see what you've got there," she said as she repositioned herself on the sofa. I handed her my résumé and photos, then I lowered myself into a mint-colored chair. She flipped cavalierly through the two pages and let them float down on the sprawling piles of papers, scripts, folders, and actor photos that hid the coffee table before relaxing back into the well-worn couch.

"Are you a gambler? Are you sick? What's wrong with you?"

This was getting uncomfortable now. "No. I'm just an actor. I do a lot of commercials right now, but I've been getting some good bit parts—like *Cheers*—lately. Why are you asking these questions?"

"Kevin," she said. She leaned forward to scrutinize me. "Kevin Sorbo." She withdrew, smiling. "I have a sense about these things, Kevin. You should be a star, and I know you will be. And I can help you do that. *If* you promise me that there's no funny business with you, that you are a normal guy—no drugs, no . . . you know—that you are who you say you are. I think great things will come your way. In fact, write down this phrase."

She rooted around the end table, found a pen in the mess there, and then ripped the blank end-page off a script near her thigh. Handing them to me, she dictated, "'Now is the time for all good men to come to the aid of their country' and sign it."

I printed as directed and signed my name below. There was something compelling about her, despite her obvious eccentricity.

I handed her the paper when I finished and sat back in my chair, waiting for—I was not sure what.

After a moment Beverlee threw her head back and laughed. "I knew it! There are great things ahead for you, Kevin Sorbo. I see it right here, in black and white. You see, I read handwriting, and yours is fantastic. Well, it's not really fantastic, because it's a bit sloppy, but that's not what I see here. I see a big career with a huge hit series. I see a lot of travel. I see you moving far away. Oh . . . never mind, you'll be back. You are going to be a huge TV star. But you won't be shooting here in LA. I'll even say you are going to the other side of the earth, like Australia or someplace, so don't be surprised."

Now it was my turn for suspicion. "Ms. Dean, are you for real?"

"Oh, don't worry, honey. I know. I freak people out a bit, but I've been doing this for ages. People, big people, powerful heads of studios, used to pay me for this stuff. The pay was good too, and I did a lot of good for them. Then one day I said something they didn't like, and now I'm living in a rent-controlled apartment instead of a Bel Air mansion. But don't worry, kiddo, I prefer working with real people—like you. And yes, what I see is real. What I see in your handwriting is golden."

"I'd like to believe that, Beverlee." I smiled at her, wondering at her sureness.

"Oh, Kevin, that's another thing. Call me Bev. We're gonna know each other a long time. Might as well make it familiar already."

SUPERMAN

IT WAS PILOT SEASON, when all the networks thrashed around, casting shows for their new fall lineups. Back then, January through April in this town was crazy. I sometimes had several auditions in a day, driving around on rain-slicked Southern California roadways, leaving plenty of time to circumvent the recent transplants from the Midwest or, worse, New Yorkers. If you couldn't afford to move to LA full time, you came for pilot season and learned to drive while finding your way to castings.

In acting classes or seminars people often state that casting agents want nothing more than to see you get the part because then their job is done. But in practice—well, let's just say, "It's complicated."

The audition process is crappy. Think *American Idol* without the immediate feedback. Although there are various ways a person becomes an agent in Hollywood, many theatrical casting agents are failed actors, putting them immediately at odds with successful ones. You never know what you might come up against in a new casting office. Casting agents can be self-assured, supportive, tough, or simply disinterested. They wield a ton of power and they know it. In general, they already have a "look" or "type" they want for a role. Sometimes the part is offered to a "star name," but maybe that person is also playing hard-to-get, so the casting agent goes through the motions of finding someone else—to motivate said name to sign on the dotted line. Politics are huge in this game, and the casting couch is still in the rotation too.

Coming from mild-mannered Minnesota, I was surprised to find Hollywood people at no loss for words when it came to judgment. They said I was too old, too young, too tall, too short (I'm six-foot-three), too muscular, too big, too insecure, too self-confident, too late, and too early. Everyone had an opinion, but the perpetual rejection only fueled my fire to prove them all wrong.

After almost seven years of kicking around LA, I was established as a working actor and had learned to navigate the turbulent and fickle audition process. When Bev called with an important audition, I was ready.

"Kevin. The studio is casting for a new show about Superman. It's perfect for you! It's got the charm of *Moonlighting* and the magic of the comic books. It's a network show, Kev."

The Man of Steel! *Now, here's a part I can really get into,* I thought.

I couldn't help myself, though, so I asked, "Do I have to wear tights?"

Bev laughed. "What? No! It's present-day!"

Lois and Clark had a great premise and a snappy script. The audition scenes (those pages are called "sides" by insiders) were witty and fun. I prepared fully, as usual. I wasn't paying for three acting classes a week and driving countless hours in rush-hour traffic to ever consider going unprepared to an audition. I arrived, signed in, and took a seat in the waiting room. There were a few guys there but no one I knew, so I sat quietly, waiting my turn and rehearsing my scenes in my head.

The casting assistant came out with an actor who was leaving and announced that we would only be reading the first scene. Typical, but I didn't begrudge them. They knew as soon as you walked in the room if they had any interest (usually not). One scene was usually enough to put any doubt to rest.

I had about a forty-five-minute wait.

Rooms can feel cold or warm, and a lot of that has to do with the casting director. They can greet you with a friendly smile or treat you with indifference, or worse. Sometimes it can be distracting when the casting director or assistant who is reading a scene with you tries to do too much with the dialogue—or too little, like not even looking at you while you're acting the scene. Today, I got lucky: Barbara Miller genuinely liked actors and enjoyed her job. She read opposite me and emoted a little as well. The entire experience was a pleasure. Plus, I was sure I nailed the reading.

At least in my mind I nailed it. Casting agents may say all sorts of things in the room, but usually they are mildly positive. Barbara thanked me for coming in with an encouraging smile, giving me the feeling that I had done well.

Not long before this audition I had reached that certain point in my career: I stopped beating myself up after castings. As long as I was happy with the way I did a scene, that was all that mattered. After an audition I would no longer get into my car and start banging on my steering wheel, cussing myself out for sucking at the audition and wishing I had done it differently. Every actor can write that same story. But about eight months before this *Superman* audition, I had made a commitment to stop doing that. And my life changed. My confidence rose, I got better feedback, and I booked more jobs. I had managed to find my peace in Hollywood—not an easy thing to do.

Sure enough, I got a callback to meet with the *Lois and Clark* producers. It was back to the Warner Bros. lot for a chance to meet the big shots at Lorimar. This was the same production company that later did the show *Friends* (you may have heard of it).

So now I was meeting Barb Miller and Les Moonves. Les has since gone on to run CBS for the last dozen years. Anyway, I nailed the reading again and was feeling pretty good.

I was called back a third time to test for the studio against four other actors. (The final audition.) My salary, and all other aspects of my potential hiring, had already been negotiated. A receptionist handed each actor our contracts for signature prior to our being allowed to enter the inner sanctum, in which, we knew, waited impatient, demanding network producers, executives, and writers. Adrenalin gripped my pen. It was nerve wracking right outside the final audition, but I also enjoyed the thrill: This was crunch time, with minutes left in the game and a tie score.

They wanted me to read opposite an actress being considered for the role of Lois. This is also typical when casting a big show, but it certainly adds to the pressure because your performance really depends a good deal on what the other person may or may not do. The chemistry between the two lead actors is important, and you have about a minute to establish some connection—anything—before beginning the scene.

I read with Teri Hatcher, who eventually earned the female lead, and they asked me to hang around in the waiting area for a bit longer afterward, together with another actor, Dean Cain. Dean and I sort of knew then that it was going to be one of us playing the Man of Steel. We both read a second time with Teri and parted ways. At that point, knowing Dean to be a strong, leading-man type, I figured we both had an equal shot at the role.

On the drive back to Santa Monica, my pager buzzed. I pulled over at the top of Barham Boulevard, the busy intersection overlooking the freeway, by a run-down liquor store that had a payphone in the parking lot. I dialed back. It was Barb Miller, who immediately congratulated me.

"Whoooohooo!" I screamed into the drone of the passing traffic. I got the part! I was stunned. I was in shock. I was actually trembling. Barb was kind on the phone, saying something like, "Well, Kevin, this is big, but you deserve it." She was genuinely happy for me. After thanking her and hanging up the phone, I looked around. These weren't the most auspicious surroundings for a life-changing experience, but they sure looked different at that moment. Everything was right with the world.

I got back in my car and let it soak in. My pager buzzed again, and I knew Barb had called Beverlee. I dialed Bev and we celebrated together with my agent, Nevin, and then I returned to my car.

I couldn't drive yet. I yelled, loudly, sitting there in my idling car. A network show, playing Superman! Then I yelled again. It was the highest high I had ever felt—higher than I got playing a varsity football or basketball game, higher than landing any role before. I was up in the clouds. How could life get any better than this?

That night, I called my parents in Minnesota and all my school friends to share the great news. It was finally sinking in, and I felt like I had arrived at the end of a long, strenuous journey. Bev had been right! (Even if her geography was off by half a world.)

I slept like a baby—once I finally could sleep—and got up early the next morning for a jog. When I got home I made scrambled eggs for breakfast, daydreaming about my promising future. Then the phone rang.

It was Barb Miller again. Very calmly, she told me the network had had a "change of heart." They were going to go with Dean Cain for the role of Clark Kent.

My body went numb as the floorboards seemed to drop out from under me. "Kevin, I'm sorry." Barb explained, embarrassed that she had apparently jumped the gun a bit by calling me the day before. "I've never seen them amend a cast decision afterward like this. They simply changed their minds." I wondered silently who the hell "they" were. She apologized profusely and reassured me I still had great promise, while my mind raced to find some reason to reject this horrible defeat. You could have drilled my healthy teeth and thrown in a few major surgeries at that moment and I wouldn't have felt a thing. In less than twenty-four hours I went from the top of Mount Everest to Hades. I was devastated. Superman was suddenly just a myth.

Not being a drinking man, I did what I always did, every day I could. I went to the gym and took all my frustrations out on the heavy steel in a mammoth workout. Then I hit the Santa Monica beach bike path and rode like a madman down to Hermosa Beach and back north to Pacific Palisades. I had to think, let off steam, and channel my frustration. This is an incredibly cruel business, from the highest of highs to the lowest of lows. I can't recommend it to anyone. But acting was my drug, so I knew I simply had to find a way to get myself out of hell and back in the game.

PAPERWORK

AT MY RIPE OLD AGE OF TEN, I have had my paper route for a year. Today I am adding a second route (my older brother's) to my delivery schedule. The alarm clock by the head of my bed rings at 4:30 A.M., but I quickly silence it. I have trained myself to rise early.

I resolutely drop my bare feet to the blue shag carpet and pull on the pair of socks I laid out the night before, careful not to wake my two older brothers, with whom I share a small room in our three-bedroom split-level. I slip on long johns and the rest of my clothes, shivering from the chilly predawn air, and I pad to our only bathroom to brush my teeth and do the rest of my morning ritual. To shake my body awake, I softly jump up and down on the frigid tiles.

My coat hangs by the front door along with my favorite blue knit hat, mittens, and scarf. I warm them up as I grab some cereal before heading outside into the frozen world.

My bicycle takes me the half-mile from my house to grab the paper drop, thinking of the newspaper truck driver who must get up even earlier than I do for his journey from Minneapolis. *He probably gets paid more too, though.*

There was no snowfall last night, but the wind is blowing gusts of it, lightly powdering everything again. The crystals on the large paper bundle immediately freeze through my mittens as I slice open its fetters, putting the folded papers in the baskets on either side of my big-wheeled bicycle. My breath is white, but the work warms my arms.

I button my jacket and jump on to start the journey to the seventy-eight houses on my route. I can do this in my sleep—and almost have. (By the time I "retire" from paper delivery, I will have executed this routine for six days a week, fifty-two weeks each year for seven years.) This morning particularly, I would rather be in bed! Winters are especially brutal in Minnesota. With the windchill, at night temperatures easily drop way below freezing, and riding my bike in the predawn hours on the icy streets puts a frost in my bones that will take hours to thaw.

As I place papers in between screen doors and big, old wooden doors, the cold starts to set in. I ride up a hill, puffing small clouds, burning my legs. My lungs start to ache from the subzero air. I try to breathe through my nose, which is running now because of the cold. My hands solidify inside their flimsy shields, frozen air passing unhindered through the knitted wool. Even my eyes are sore, blinking against the wind.

On the way back down the hill, I ball my hands into fists, needing only small pushes to steer the bike that is virtually an extension of my body. I am more than halfway there, about to start my new second route.

I battle the cold with frozen resolve, and I finish.

Once home, I hastily drop my bike in the garage and head inside to change out of my long johns and grab some breakfast before school. First, I pump my fists to return the blood flow and speed the heat there. The feeling in my fingers slowly comes back, and I can unbutton my shirt.

Early in my life I began nurturing my sense of responsibility and a hearty determination to overcome anything that got in my way.

HALF-GOD

THREE MONTHS HAD PASSED, and I was still feeling the intense rejection from the whole Superman incident. I knew this was part of my business, but sometimes the self-pity could just pile up and wear me down.

Nevin, my agent, called. "Kevin, Nevin here. I have a role that is perfect for you. It is a TV movie about Hercules—four of them, actually. I am sending the script to your apartment now. Check it out and tell me what you think."

Hercules? From Superman to this? I laughed. I was a reasonably big guy, a tad over six-foot-three and 220 pounds at the time, but I figured they would need a guy who was 280 pounds of no-neck steroids to play the legendary half god–half mortal, the strongest man in the world. I thought about it for a while and then picked up the phone to chat with Beverlee. "I was just going to call you!" Although she didn't exactly scream, she always had full-on cheerleader enthusiasm (just add megaphone).

"Bev, really? First Superman and now a Greek god? I am not in the mood to go through this, especially since you know they want some body-builder-on-the-beach dude. I'll be wasting my time."

Beverlee kept her cool. "Kevin, I read the script. You will love this. Just go in there and do what you do. Universal is planning on shooting four made-for-TV Hercules movies, and they are going to New Zealand! Remember what I told you when we first met? I told you Australia, I know.

New Zealand is close enough, though. I am right about these things, Kevin. I know."

Silence. Deep breath. "Sure, Bev." I said. "I will go in there and kick some butt."

The actors in the waiting room at Universal Studios in Burbank ranged from skinny, wimpy dudes to guys much bigger than me. That gave me a little relief, actually, because I could see the studio didn't even know what it wanted for this part. I determined to do my best with the sides (script pages) that, though no great tribute to Shakespeare, were meaty enough to dig my teeth into.

There were two scenes, and they asked me to read both of them. That was a good sign, so as I drove home after the audition, I called manager and agent, told them it went well, and then forgot about it. As usual, it was a crapshoot.

Two weeks later I got a callback. Callbacks indicate you've done something right. I showed up early at the same casting office, only to discover even more actors of every type waiting to audition, and no one I recognized from before. Clearly, they had no idea what they were look-ing for, but at least I was still in the running. My confidence intact, I per-formed the sides again, said thanks, and left.

I got another callback a few weeks later, then another one a few weeks after that. This went on for almost three months. Usually by the third callback you are testing for studio executives. After that it starts feeling weird. I had six callbacks on this role, and during the last two, the room was filled to capacity with all the studio and producer suits, but we still had not negotiated any contract. I was frustrated and sure I was wasting my time. "I see the script hasn't changed, but is there something you'd like me to do differently this time?" I asked politely. One of the produc-ers answered, "No, no, Kevin. You're great. We liked what you did before; we just need to see it again." It began to seem like an elaborate hoax—perhaps there was no role at all.

Months after my first audition for the role, we negotiated a deal. That seemed like progress—finally. The seventh audition was the studio test, with signed contracts. There were five of us still in the running, which had been narrowed down from the initial 2,500 who auditioned. After I performed the sides, a female executive suggested that it might be good if they could see me without my shirt on to see what kind of shape I was in. I made some flirtatious joke about a woman wanting to see me with my shirt off and asked all the men to leave the room. They all laughed— and stayed. My physique was my most obvious asset, especially in the commercial world, so I was not shy about my body. When the shirt came off I could see a uniformly happy reaction from the ten nicely dressed executives, but it did feel strange to be the only shirtless man in the room!

"Would you be willing to shave your chest and stomach?" one of the producers asked. I am not hirsute, but I do have "man cover" on my front. I told him I would consider it. "Although, I don't think Hercules would have been clean shaven," I pointed out. "I mean, when would he have had the time for personal grooming?" More laughter. Then they all thanked me and I left.

For days I heard nothing—not a peep—and no one knew anything when I called for feedback. After several days I let it go entirely. That's show business.

A few weeks later, on September 24, Bev and Nevin conference called to wish me a happy birthday. I was in Vancouver, British Columbia, filming a guest spot on the set of Stephen Cannell's series *The Commish*.

"We have a special birthday present for you, Kevin." Nevin sounded nonchalant, as usual.

"Oh, really?" I answered. "What is it?"

"You, my friend," countered Bev, "are the world's next Hercules!"

The phone was silent for what seemed like a very long time.

"Kevin?" Bev asked tentatively. "Are you there?"

Then that buzz surged through my veins again. I let out a solid yell. "Whooo-hooo!" They laughed.

"Now what? What's the next step?" I asked, half afraid that this too would vanish the next day.

"You start training the day you get back from Vancouver, so get ready," Nevin said. "You will be training with Douglas Wong, one of Bruce Lee's original students, for all the martial arts and fight prep. And you'll also do some intensive horseback riding work. This is going to be part of Universal's "Action Pack," Kevin. They have four other shows they will be shooting at the same time, packaging them all together in a rotation of airings on TV. Trust me, this is big! It's a new genre: action television. The studio is really going to promote these. Congratulations."

"It's perfect for you!" Bev added. I was smiling big. A year in New Zealand. I got the part!

I walked back on the set of *The Commish* and looked around. Nothing had changed, but everything looked different to me.

American shows filmed almost exclusively in the United States and Canada. I reflected on Bev's unlikely prediction with awe and a new sense of appreciation for her. When I got back to LA I was booked into a six-week Action Hero Boot Camp, and the rest, as they say, is history— with a little mythology thrown in.

After a thirteen-hour plane ride, I arrived early on November 5 in Auckland, New Zealand. Tremendous turbulence had thrashed the plane over the Pacific, so I was tired (I have never slept well on planes) but still totally stoked to be in a new country, ready for a new adventure. As I walked to the baggage claim area, birds sang on a repeating recording. It was cheerful and guileless, and it made me smile.

Auckland airport, situated outside the city amongst the sheep and cow pastures, was single-level and just large enough to handle the jumbo planes of the long international flights servicing the country. How small, you ask? My producer Eric Gruendemann had parked in the pick-up lane of the airport.

Eric was a tall, relaxed guy with thick brown hair and an easy smile. This was our first meeting in person. He offered to take one of my bags, saying, "The car isn't far. Is this all the luggage you have? You should show my wife how to pack. We brought the kitchen sink!"

We emerged into broken sunshine and a double rainbow in the distance. "See what I arranged for your arrival? Now, don't say I never did anything for you." He chuckled at his own joke while I marveled at my incredible luck.

"Thanks," I said, as I grabbed my camera from my carry-on and took a shot. "Hey, maybe you should get second unit out here and shoot this for stock footage."

"Not to worry, you'll see plenty of rainbows while you are here," he said.

I walked over to the sedan and we found ourselves standing on the same side of the car. He gave me a wry look. "What, you think you're okay to drive already?"

"What? Oh!" In New Zealand they drive on the left side of the road, so the driver's side of the car is on the right. "You know, you're right. I am a little too tired to drive right now. But thanks for offering."

Eric had a sarcastic sense of humor, like mine. We were destined to be good friends.

At our first cast read-through in Auckland I met Michael Hurst, who was to play Hercules's sidekick, Iolaus. I had been told he was a serious theater actor, seasoned and very talented. Our over nine-inch height difference was the first thing anyone noticed. Michael immediately started making jokes about needing to walk on boxes or stilts on the set. His commentary reflected the nervous energy in the room. We were all charting new waters with this project, embarking simultaneously on a new movie and entertainment genre. (*Hercules* was part of Universal Studio's "Action Pack," a collection of five action-filled dramatic productions.) Would it work or flop?

Our foreign element also added to the tension in the room. Roma Downey (a recent Emmy winner who went on to *Touched by an Angel*), Eric Gruendemann, Bill Norton (the director), Anthony Quinn, and I represented the minority but dominant nation on the project. Sure, New Zealand had hosted other TV and movie productions before, but this was a massive effort from a powerful American studio. Although the locals sometimes resented the great shadow the US cast, everyone understood this was a chance to put the Kiwi film industry on the map professionally. (Years later Michael told me that his theater friends gave him crap for "caving in" and accepting a part on an American TV show. I asked him who, and he laughed, saying, "I can't tell you because they've all come in to guest star on the show!")

As much as I liked the first script, it bothered me that the Hercules character was such a serious guy and a self-absorbed womanizer with a violent streak. He was so unlikeable, it was almost silly. I worried that people wouldn't want to watch the show, so I bent the ears of the producers. "Guys, the audience is either going to laugh at us or with us. I think we want them laughing with us." I started by throwing in some off-hand jokes, knowing that if the studio didn't approve, they could always edit them out. They stayed in. Michael and I, with Eric Gruendemann's blessing, played off each other on set, adding more humor—a lot more humor. The writers back home in the States picked up on that and started writing more comical scenes. It was goofy but fun, which is what made *Hercules: The Legendary Journeys* so enjoyable for so many, including us on set.

During the filming of the second movie, *Hercules and the Underworld*, Michael Hurst and I really found our groove. We talked a lot on set and determined that the magic of our relationship lay in being the Butch and Sundance of our imaginary millennium. For example, there was one particular scene in which Hercules and Iolaus are being chased by an angry mob because Hercules has been framed for murders that he didn't commit. The angry mob is circling the inn where we are "holed up" and we have to make our escape. As Michael and I run through a doorway, Michael has his bow accidentally turned horizontal, and of course, he bounces right back into me. It was a genius accident. Everyone cracked up, and we kept it in the scene. Many things like this had been happening over the previous month, just clicking into place, creating the right amount of humor to mix with the drama, but that was the exact moment I knew.

I called Beverlee that night. "Bev, Universal is going to make *Hercules* a weekly series!"

"What?!" she yelled. "Who told you that? No one called me."

"Trust me. I just know it, Bev. We have hit our stride and it feels great!" Within the week a fifth movie was added to the schedule, and within the month the studio decreed we would go straight into a one-hour series. That was fine by me. (Although initially the studio considered *Hercules* the least viable of the five members of the "Action Pack," only *Vanishing*

Son accompanied us into episodic production. Unfortunately, they were canceled the following year.)

By the time we graduated into shooting the series, our set worked like a Swiss movement. The camera crew was a tight team and ready to roll. The main actors were thoroughly prepared and our relationships were solid. My costume had gone from a dark linen vest to yellow chamois (contrasting better with the fake tan), and my woven leather pants were also better fitted. The best part was that my hair had grown out enough to remove the annoying hair extensions I had needed for the first year of filming. We continued working a grueling schedule of six-day weeks, but because everyone had a lot of fun and none of us knew how long the good times would last, no one complained. This was the first big Hollywood production in New Zealand, employing at once about two hundred people, and that was just for starters. It was a boon to the economy and to the artistic and production communities, which would eventually create all the *Lord of the Rings* movies and more. Many of the Oscar winners from those movies got their start on the set of *Hercules*.

Personally, I loved to work—to excess. My schedule was insane, although at the time it was simply what I did. I hit the floor running at about 4:30 every morning. I took a quick wake-up shower and stretched to warm up for the fight scenes that awaited, made oatmeal or a smoothie, and jumped in the car. I was usually one of the first people on set at about 6:30, and catering would make me another breakfast, eggs this time. Our makeup artist Annie did makeup and hair like a virtuoso playing "London Bridge." I'd put on my costume and go back for my fake tan, which Annie unceremoniously slapped on, using big floppy sponges. We called it "Spartacus Sheen." My boots together with the woven leather pants weighed twelve pounds, and a costume assistant laced them for me. Not until the start of season three did I get smart enough to suggest they put real running-shoe insoles into the boots for my poor feet, so those suckers were about as real as they looked on screen. (Now, three knee surgeries later, I'm glad I at least spoke up when I did!)

About twice a week the shoot day included a long session of choreography to learn the fight sequence. Our stunt coordinator, Peter Bell, was an amazingly creative and proficient designer, and he was a hair stylist on the side! He could kick butt and look good doing it, I guess.

Yes, back then I did all my own fights and every stunt the producers allowed me to do. I was dedicated and athletic, and I was too proud to allow someone else to double me. In fact, in the opening credits of the show there is a shot of the back of a Hercules body double, walking. It bugs me to this day because, frankly, he isn't walking in character!

The fights were long and involved, as Peter and I always wanted to outdo what we had done before. The stunt men he hired, "stuntees," were awesome, doing backflips from my fake hits. We trained hard and rehearsed those fights over and over before shooting them. It is truly the only way to love your job: keep challenging yourself to do better. Too often these days fight scenes are shot with lots of smoke and fast cuts, and they are unclear and confusing. With only hours to shoot our fights, we got better looking footage than some movies that take days for their sequences, and that is a testament to Peter Bell, the stunt team, and John Mahaffie, our director of photography.

One of the coolest things we did was rig our guys on wires, so when I pretended to hit them, they flew thirty feet through the air and made it look realistic—or at least really awesome. More than once I lifted a guy across both my shoulders and spun around, "hitting" various stuntees who fell away as if irreparably injured.

All of that made for long, exhausting days, and at the end of each day, around 7:30 in the evening, we would wrap on set and I'd drive myself to the Les Mills Gym.

Les Mills was a longtime New Zealand athlete and Olympic competitor. After retiring from competition he became a gym owner and businessman, also serving as Auckland's mayor for almost a decade. The gym he named for himself was the hangout for anyone serious about either working out or appearing to work out. I was friendly with a lot of the patrons, but I did have a couple of crazy stalker-types show up there to meet me. They were harmless enough. (The only one who really freaked me out was the woman who tracked me down at home. I had disclosed in an interview that I lived on a lake. She found the biggest lake near Auckland and apparently talked to enough neighbors to knock on my door at midnight one night. There she was, slightly creepy, carefully dressed, perspiring from running around in heels, and smiling at me in the dim light of my front porch. She introduced herself and offered me a "massage." I kindly refused her generous proposal. Visibly disappointed and irritated, she left in a huff.)

The show was wildly popular—we could see that in the ratings and reviews—but distance insulated me. Sure, I was getting invites to premieres and parties back in Los Angeles and New York, but I could never attend because I was a world away. Paparazzi didn't hound me on the streets in New Zealand—they didn't really exist there. As peculiar as it was, a doorstep massage offer was my closest call with stardom thus far.

After a day on set I would spend about two hours at the gym. I was lifting really heavily back then, benching 325 and feeling very manly. That got me home at around ten. A quick shower and some dinner, and I was ready to study my lines before crashing at midnight. My head would hit the pillow and I'd be out like an exploded light bulb. I didn't dream. Then the alarm would sound immediately (at 4:30 A.M. once more), leaving me feeling like I had slept only five minutes. It was like I shut down for four and a half hours to recharge my batteries for the next day.

For the first two years of the show that was my schedule, six days each week. Before season three the producers figured out that the schedule was murder. (I told them they were killing me.) The following season they lightened the schedule to five-day weeks. This gave me extra time to do interviews and work on the scripts on Saturdays, but I also finally had time to play golf again, which made me very happy.

⌒

I have been in Auckland for only about four months. We are shooting the third movie, which is big news in the small country.

This guy walks up to me in the gym as I am doing a set of curls, sizes me up, and says, "You're that Yankee shooting that show *Hercules*, eh?" (Add Kiwi accent for flavor.)

I finish my set and put down my weights. I know where this is going.

"Yep," I say.

"American, eh?"

"Yep," I say.

He gives me full-on attitude and says, "Well I've been to America. *Hated* it."

Don't bother going back, then. We've got enough assholes there already, I'm thinking, but I just smile to myself and nod. Specifically in a gym, there's something provocative about being the guy who plays Hercules; lots of times when I'm working out, I can feel the eyes on me. Most people who come up to me are excited or fans of the show and say so, but there are always those dudes who are less enthusiastic to see me.

One Christmas I'm home in Minneapolis visiting my mom and dad. A new gym has opened up, so I get a week's pass. I'm on the bench press about to lift the barbell off the rack, and these two pretty big guys walk by, whispering—snickering.

"I can lift more than that," one says, loud enough for me to hear. Then, "Wimp."

Good Lord, I say to myself. *I'm in my thirties, these guys are in their thirties, and it's like we're in high school.* The gym brings out people's insecurities, I guess.

Another time I'm working out at Gold's Gym in Henderson, Nevada, before I head off to promote *Kull*. An average guy in a faded red baseball cap—maybe five-foot-seven, 150 pounds—swaggers up to me and says, "Hey, you're Kevin Sorbo!"

"Yes, I am. Nice to meet you."

He is in no particular shape, with some mild definition in his arms and the start of a beer belly. He looks me up and down and, without even cracking a smile, says, "Damn, I thought you'd be bigger. I should have auditioned for that part!"

Seriously?

Having been in this situation more often than you might guess, I have developed a few clever answers to comments like, "I thought you'd be bigger."

"Why, thank you."

"And I thought you'd be better looking."

And my all-time favorite: "Well, I am *huge* from the waist down."

PRINCE HERCULES

MY ENTIRE NEW ZEALAND SOCIAL LIFE was on set or the occasional poker night with—who else?—people from the set: my costar, Michael; my producer, Eric; and some stuntees, makeup artists, cameramen, or even an occasional guest star. I was alone, save for what my work provided. I was not integrated into the town of Auckland—there was no time for that. I did not have a love life—how could I? I stayed in touch with family and friends back home by phone, but only occasionally. My schedule and the time difference conspired against me.

I have always loved traveling to different places; the restless gypsy in me forever searching for that next adventure. I just needed to keep going. Keep experiencing. Keep escaping from some unseen force I felt was chasing me and trying to get me to *stop* running. Even the firm commitment of the TV show was, in fact, a limited time frame, which was fine by me. That meant my options stayed open. The idea of "settling" was a difficult pill to swallow, and I had slowly but agreeably resigned myself to being a bachelor for the rest of my life. This wasn't a sad admission. It was just a fact.

Nearly every episode of *Hercules* called for a new guest star, and 99 percent of them were female. Nice working environment, if you know what

I mean—I am the first to admit I am an inveterate flirt. (Come on, now—it's just good sport!)

I always promised that when I had my own show, I would call up every guest star ahead of time to make them feel welcome, and I made good on that. There can be enormous egos on TV sets, and the week's guest star is the odd man out, especially in a new country. I wanted to put them at ease.

To play the part of Princess Kirin in an upcoming episode, the producers cast an actress named Sam Jenkins. *That's a great name for such a babe*, I thought as I looked at her photo. (Since my pre-teenage crush on the gorgeous Bobbie Jo Bradley of *Petticoat Junction*, I've been a fan of guys' names on pretty girls.) Sam would be playing my love interest in episode forty-nine, almost four years into the show's production. In early June of 1996 I made my introductory call to her in her apartment.

"Hi, Sam. I'm Kevin Sorbo from *Hercules*."

The air was dead, so I continued. "You're coming down to guest star on the show."

"Oh, yes, I know! Sorry! You caught me completely off guard." There was a soft, unexpected intimacy in her voice. "Hi! How are you?"

"I'm fine, thanks. I'm just calling to welcome you to the show. I know it's a long way to travel, so I wanted you to know we are happy you are coming."

"Wow. This is a first. It's so nice of you to call. Um, thanks!"

"No problem. I just want you to feel comfortable. You're going to enjoy New Zealand. It's a beautiful country."

"Well, it's already full of surprises, that's for sure!" She sounded so happy, giddy—it was infectious. "I'm, uh, looking forward to meeting you in person. You have a great voice, but you've probably heard that before. Is there anything you'd like me to bring you from the States?"

A future costar had never asked me that before. "Oh, thanks. That's nice of you to offer, but I'm good here."

"Yep, that's what I've heard . . ."

What? Was she flirting with me? I laughed. *She's stealing my moves.*

"I'm sorry. I can't believe I just said that," she said. "I'm just having fun with you."

"Well, don't stop on my account!" I answered. She laughed. I could tell we were going to have some fun together.

Our first scene fell on a Friday, and afterward we went to a production dinner at my favorite restaurant. Although our group was over a dozen people, I talked almost exclusively with Sam all dinner long. I was totally enthralled. The next day I took my brother and his son skiing on the South Island for the weekend as we had planned. I had invited Sam and her sister to join us, but they said they were content to experience Auckland instead. It made sense, but it was strangely disappointing for me. That weekend I inexplicably found myself daydreaming of Sam and white picket fences. I couldn't get her out of my mind. I didn't want to, either.

Monday, on set, I began my pursuit in earnest. Sam was smart and funny and beautiful, and most intriguing: She was only mildly receptive to my advances. (How she could resist me, I'll never know, but I was determined to wear her down.) I asked her out on a date the following Saturday.

We got to the movie early and sat in the empty theater chatting about our lives and our dreams. Somehow I found myself discussing my future children. "Since high school I've had a vision that's always stuck with me. I just knew I would have three kids in the order boy, boy, girl. Funny, the things we latch onto as children," I mused.

Sam looked at me earnestly and smiled, saying, "That's what I'm having too, in that order. I've known it all my life."

I laughed. We talked some more, and I can't possibly explain how it came up, but I confessed to her that I planned to get married in a small chapel in the Alps. "I was there on a modeling assignment out of Munich. It's beautiful, sitting on a gentle hilltop surrounded by towering mountains. It's very romantic."

"Wait a minute," she said warily. "In Garmisch?"

I swallowed, "That's the one." *She knew the town? She knew the place?*

"Yeah, okay, you better stop now," she protested, putting her finger up as a warning, "because you're really starting to freak me out." That was her dream wedding chapel as well.

After that our mutual attraction was undeniable. On set, I would take Sam's hand to gently lead her behind the scenery, and I would just kiss her. It hit me so quickly and so hard, the idea that I had found *the one*— and after I had finally given up. I pursued her with everything I had. It was just the way I lived: fast paced, on the edge, fully invested.

The episode we met on, *Prince Hercules*, is one of my favorite episodes. I shot another *Hercules* episode after Sam wrapped and then had to rush off to Bratislava, Slovakia, to shoot *Kull, the Conqueror*. I stopped in Los Angeles on the way to do the *Tonight Show* and a few other publicity bookings and was able to see Sam there. I invited her to visit me in Slovakia and she accepted, even though she was shooting a recurring part on *Chicago Hope* at the time. She said she would find a way to work it out with her producers.

While I was in Europe shooting *Kull* I got a call from Rob Tapert, the executive producer of *Hercules*, saying they wanted to write a three-show arc about a half deer–half woman that Hercules falls in love with. Rob mentioned that the chemistry between Sam and me looked great on film and asked if I would mind working with her again for six weeks. Wary of showing too much enthusiasm, I feigned disinterest, saying, "Yeah, she was okay. I think she would be a good choice."

I hung up the phone and immediately called Sam with the exciting news. Those six weeks of shooting leading up to the Christmas season, with Sam playing the Golden Hind character, solidified our relationship. I asked her to move down to Auckland so we could be together, but she wanted the whole deal: a ring and a date.

Surprising even myself, I was willing to go along with that. I proposed in early January. We were engaged within six months of meeting each other.

And we had plans for a family: boy, boy, girl.

Though I had finally found the love of my life, I still maintained the eternal love affair with my job, my character, and the show. Old habits die hard. Every day on set offered a new opportunity to hone my skills and advance my craft, to learn from the generous and talented crew surrounding me, to create, and to entertain. I was blindly and resolutely devoted to my work, neglecting almost everything else life offered. My every moment was accounted for and committed, and I liked it that way. I had everything I believed I needed, and it demanded all of me. When I was offered a feature film over my hiatus from the show, I grabbed the chance without a thought that it would mean absolutely no vacation or downtime at all. Far from a change of pace, the film work was equally grueling, with huge fight scenes and long hours on set in a foreign country that offered few social distractions. After finishing, it was right back to the *Hercules* schedule. I couldn't complain; it was everything I loved. I was chasing my dreams and realizing them.

But after four years of that intense, grueling schedule, my body had maxed out all of its reserves. Outwardly, I had reached a pinnacle of physical, emotional, and professional success.

Inside, however, my body was about to betray me.

THE VOICE

THE THIRD OF SEPTEMBER 1997 was another beautiful sunny day in Southern California. After touring eight cities in seven days to promote my feature film *Kull: The Conqueror*, doing interviews, and making appearances signing autographs morning, noon, and night, I had a day free from publicists and producers. Though I was certainly feeling like I was on top of the world—hit TV show, my first major motion picture just opening and another set to start shooting in two weeks—some troublesome issues preoccupied me.

For the previous several months my left arm and hand had been intermittently painful, aching, tingling, cold, and numb. I had assumed it would just clear up on its own, but the problem had gradually gotten worse. Several doctors at various hotels on my publicity tour thought it was not serious. I even had what seemed like a rational explanation: I had injured my ulnar nerve, or funny bone. Why should I question them? And yet, today, my arm was really bugging me. So I did what felt best. I went to the gym, of course.

I needed to clear my head and work off some of my irritation, but I didn't get very far. After a good long cardio I picked up some free weights for bicep curls. Searing pain shot down from my left shoulder, hurting so much I actually had to put down the weights.

Now I was really peeved. I had grown up playing golf, football, basketball, and baseball. As a former football defensive end, let's just say it takes a lot of punishment before I call it quits. During my senior year, in the first football game of the season, I took a lot of hard hits. One opposing player got his helmet under mine, into my chin. After the play I went to the sideline so full of adrenaline that I didn't even know I had split my chin open so far that people could see bone. That was the third time for me for that particular football injury. The team medic did a quick tape-up on the sidelines. Later in that game I got nailed from the side, helmet to helmet, and the combination of the shoulder pads and helmets just wiped me out, resulting in a pinched nerve that lasted not only through the rest of that football season but also most of basketball season as well. I played through that brutal pain because it was the only way I would get to play. I had never just quit—until now.

From the corner of my eye I saw my old friend Charles Glass training a client. Charles had been a presence at Gold's for as long as I had been there, and he was in perfect physical condition. It aggravated me to watch him work when I couldn't pick the five-pounder up off the rack.

"Hey, Kev, how's it going?" he asked amiably.

"Good, good, but I'm done now," I answered, not willing to admit defeat, even to myself.

I left the gym. My chiropractor of eight years was on the west side of town—close enough to Gold's. I phoned him. "I need to see the doc, today, if possible. I've got some intense shoulder pain, tingling in my fingers, and they feel cold too."

The receptionist told me to come in that afternoon. I ran to my favorite eatery, The Omelet Parlor. This establishment has been in Venice since 1977, and although it's a bit timeworn, with cheap wood paneling and stained floral wallpaper, I love the old black-and-white beach photos that adorn its walls. They recall an earlier generation, with women clad in swim-dresses with parasols and the men in union suits and caps, lounging on the undeveloped raw shoreline that currently hosts towering condos, hotels, restaurants, and parking lots. I ruminated on the passage of time and downed a quick lunch before heading over to see the doc.

I liked coming to Doctor Hank's airy second-story office because of the Zen ambiance. There was a large, wispy fern in the corner next to a bubbling stone fountain. A framed print of a brook sloshing languidly over moss-covered rocks hung behind the small, wooden reception desk. Midday sunlight filtered in through the bamboo blinds, glinting off the dust that hovered in the still air.

Dr. Hank invited me into his office. He was quiet and reserved. I always relaxed under his care, and I was looking for some of that today. He examined my arm with a frown, and then noticed a lump on the top of my shoulder, which he prodded a bit. It was soft but immovable. I lay down on his table and he proceeded to twist my spine and stretch my arms and legs to adjust my alignment. Then he moved up to my head and started massaging my neck. He had sure, capable hands, and I immediately felt the tension start to fade.

Then I heard a voice: *"Don't let him crack your neck."*

"What did you say?" I asked him, mystified. The first time Doctor Hank adjusted my neck, about eight years earlier, I told him I didn't like it. I thought we had an implicit agreement that he would never try it again.

"I didn't say anything," Doctor Hank replied easily, "but I was just going to comment that you've got a lot of tightness in your neck and shoulders." His practiced hands continued to massage my neck, relieving some of my headache as my stress dissipated.

"Oh, okay," I said. He had gotten me completely relaxed, which is why I had come here.

"Don't let him crack your neck."

I heard that soft yet powerful voice again. Disturbing. I wondered why I was hearing these words in my head. Doctor Hank never did that, anyway.

Then he jerked my head to the side. *Click! Crack! Pop!* I jumped up to sitting and looked at him, rubbing my neck.

"Why . . . why did you do that?" I demanded.

"I just felt that you needed it. Your neck was really bad." I felt flushed and a little light-headed, so I looked around, stretching my neck in different directions. It seemed okay.

"You never do that," I chided, perplexed by my anger. I calmed down and reasoned with myself. It really wasn't a big deal, after all: just a quick crack and I was fine. But that voice had warned me against it, and I just knew something was wrong.

"Sorry if it startled you, but you really did need it. That should feel much better now. As for the lump on your shoulder, I'm afraid I'm stumped. You may want to get your internist to check that for you."

I was preoccupied with that voice in my head. It seemed conspicuously silent.

The receptionist was back. I paid the bill she laid on the counter and went out to my rental car. I got inside my Jeep Cherokee, put on the tunes, and headed down toward Wilshire Boulevard. I turned left to go to my fiancée Sam's Beverly Hills condo, listening to Journey's "Don't Stop Believing," even singing along. I love that song. I had no idea, of course, how significant it would prove.

About five minutes went by before everything went haywire, like bad static on a TV.

An electric pulse got stuck inside my brain and ricocheted around for what felt like a small eternity. It was like a blow to the head: confusion, at first. In situations like this, you don't really know exactly what's happened until you're able to focus, which was what I tried to do. I didn't panic at that point. I was still trying to put the sensation into perspective, into past tense. But it wasn't going away.

I felt sick to my stomach, like after a bad rollercoaster ride. Startled and woozy, I somehow managed to maneuver the Jeep safely to the side of the road, trembling violently, hitching my breaths. I sat in the car for about a minute, or maybe ten—who was counting? An 8.9 earthquake had struck my head and I was still having aftershocks. Finally, the intense electric zapping in my brain subsided, but my head was still buzzing. I realized I was hyperventilating. That's when the panic burst in.

My heart was racing. I hardly recognized my white-knuckled hands gripping the steering wheel. "No," I said, willing my body to pay attention, forcing my hands to release, splaying my fingers like a child.

"Wait a sec, wait a sec, wait a minute . . . and let's see, okay, okay, let's see what's going on." I put the car in park and then breathed through my nose and tensed my arms and legs to control the shaking. I looked out the window at the passing cars, blurred projectiles that shimmered like a school of fish. I was spinning and wobbling, like a top in its death throes. *What just happened? And what was still happening?*

Slowly, I calmed. I phoned Sam. "Hi. Um, listen, I went to Doctor Hank, and I'm on Wilshire now, and I feel really strange. Like my head is inside an aquarium and I am looking out through the water and glass. I can't see right. Everything is kind of blurry. I'm shivering too."

"What happened?" she asked. I wanted to be calm, but the panic in my voice resonated in my clenched gut. Deep breath in.

"I don't know. I was just driving and I felt this . . . jolt. This really big jolt, like an electric shock in my brain. Now everything is—at a distance, like I can't focus on it, like I'm inside an aquarium."

"Should I come get you?"

Talking was helping me, but inside, my stomach was a solid block of granite. "No, wait, Sam, listen. It was so weird, because right before he cracked my neck, I heard a voice tell me not to let him."

"A voice?"

"Sam, I'm telling you, this voice said, 'Don't let him crack your neck,' clear as day, inside my head. Twice. I think I really screwed up. I don't know."

"No, honey, I'm sure you didn't. But then you let him crack your neck anyway?"

"I had no idea he would—he never, ever does. But today he did. And now this really weird thing just happened, and it's . . . shit, Sam . . ."

"Okay, pull over. I mean, stay there. Tell me where you are, and I'll come pick you up." Her voice was soothing and insistent.

But I didn't want her to have to come out to get me. I was a hardened thirty-eight, not an eleven-year-old, after all. "No, no, I'm okay." I stalled for a few minutes, trying to get my head back to normal, willing it to just kick in, like trying to start a car with a dead battery. I could hear my brain engine trying to turn over. *Rrrr-rrrr-rrrrr.* It wouldn't engage.

This was ridiculous, and I wasn't going to cave in to whatever it was. I did feel more focused by now, too. "You know, I feel a little bit better. I'll keep driving. I'm okay to drive home."

"Kevin, you don't sound like you are. Let me come get you. Where exactly are you?"

"Wait, no . . . I'm okay to drive home. I just don't feel well. I'm kind of nauseated too. It was the strangest thing to feel, Sam. But I'm a bit better now. I'm back on the road. I'm not far away even."

"Okay, I'll stay on the phone with you till you get here, 'kay?" Sam sounded unconvinced, but she was a team player, and I was captain of this game, anyway. She had no idea what was going on in my head. Frankly, neither did I. I was in fight mode, and I just wanted to get home. I didn't realize then that my body—my brain—was already locked in the battle for my life.

Sam stayed on the phone with me until I was about half a mile away, and she was waiting at the door for me when I came in. It wasn't quite three in the afternoon. We had a 4:30 P.M. pick-up for a taping of *The Vibe*, a TV talk show produced by Quincy Jones over at CBS West Hollywood. I was their main guest, and I'd be leaving them high and dry if I didn't show up.

"I don't think I can go," I said. "I really don't feel well." I went into the bedroom to lie down. Sam called the chiropractor to see if maybe he knew what I was reacting to, but he had no idea.

Sam scrutinized my face. "Should I take you to the hospital? Is it that bad?"

"No, no hospital." I was an athlete. I didn't like hospitals. "It's not that bad, but it's bad. I can't explain it, I just feel really sick, but in a different way than sick sick, you know?"

"Not really," she answered, "but if you want, I'll call Peg and cancel for you."

Peg, the tireless publicist, wouldn't take kindly to a cancellation, especially at the last minute. But two hours' notice was better than a moment's.

Peg was horrified on the phone. "Oh, crap, Kevin, you just can't do this to them, with only an hour till taping. I mean, what's wrong with you, actually? Are you injured?"

She was freaking out. I couldn't explain myself any better, and frankly, I was too exhausted to try anyway. Not wanting to disappoint anyone, I decided to take a rest and try my damndest to get there. I fell asleep.

Peg was genuinely thrilled to see us arrive in the town car at the appointed time. Sam and I went backstage to my room and waited for them to call me. Beverlee was already there, smiling through a worried look. Bev knew me to fight through anything, so my call trying to beg off the show must have thrown her for a loop. I mumbled something reassuring to her about a bad headache and powered through as best I could.

I do not remember what we discussed on the show, but it must have been an interview about *Kull*. Because I had done so many already, I was on autopilot, even though the entire world was spinning. The audience was too loud, and my head was throbbing, pounding, splitting—you name it. It could not have ended soon enough, and we took off back home immediately after.

As we walked out to the car, with me holding on to Sam, we bumped into an old friend I hadn't seen in a while. My head was now on fire. I tried to make small talk, to be cool and look like all was well, but it was a brutal battle to hold it all together.

Thus began the best acting of my life—acting like I was healthy.

The following morning, a determined sun streaked in around the closed curtains. It was early yet and the world was fuzzy and unfixed. I still felt the loud buzzing in my head, so I relented and took some more Ibuprofen. I had never been a pill-popper, eschewing medicines for a revitalizing jog or workout when I had a cold or aches. In the past few days I had taken more Ibuprofen than I had in my entire life up to that point.

I got some breakfast and turned on the TV. It was too loud, so I turned it down—all the way—and just sank into the couch and stared at the moving pictures. What was going on? Why wouldn't this dizziness go away? Why did everything seem blurry?

I called my internist as soon as his office opened. They gave me an appointment for that morning.

I laced up my Nikes, kissed Sam goodbye, and headed off for a long walk to Dr. Huizenga's office. After what had happened yesterday, I didn't trust myself driving. Sam had offered to take me the mile and a half, but

I hoped the fresh morning air would help clear my head and reset my energy level. By the time I got there I was feeling slightly better. Any small improvement was encouraging.

Dr. Robert Huizenga is kind of a celebrity doctor in Hollywood. Currently, his claim to fame is *The Biggest Loser*, other TV appearances, and several books. An alumnus of Harvard Medical School, he was team physician for the Oakland Raiders for several years. He knows athletes, and he is one himself. In fact, he works out daily, does not put on body fat, and does not age. Honestly, I suspect he's a cyborg, but this was no time for jokes.

I told Dr. Rob everything that had happened. My arm was now the least of my concerns. He put me through some neurological tests: standing on one foot and walking the tightrope, one foot in front of the other. He had me touch my nose and then his finger, each time moving his finger for me to follow. I did not perform as well as I should have—or at least as well as I expect out of myself. I have a fast reaction time, and I felt like I was moving through molasses.

Dr. Rob puzzled over my cold, numb fingers. He put my arm through its range of motion and did a cursory overall physical exam. "I don't like this lump in your shoulder," he said. "I can make some guesses at what it is, but that wouldn't be too professional, now would it?" In spite of his light tone, I saw concern on his face.

"So what do you want to do?" I asked.

"Let's set up a biopsy later this week. It's a sensitive area, so it needs to be done in the hospital."

I had to digest this information. "What about my eyesight?" I asked. "I am having trouble focusing; I have this weird kind of blind spot happening."

He slowed. "You see Dr. Castor, right?" Castor had performed corrective surgery on my eyes years before, freeing me from glasses. I nodded. "Let's get you over there right now and have him check that out. I'll call him and let him know you're on your way."

Castor's office was only four blocks from Dr. Rob's, so I walked directly there. Outside in the breezy daylight, I felt better.

Dr. Castor quietly and methodically performed a full eye exam. This included a sight test, in which I stared at a center light and then tapped a button when I saw a pinpoint of light flash in my periphery.

"I cannot explain why your eyesight was blurry but isn't anymore today, Kevin," Dr. Castor said somberly. "You do have a roughly 15 percent vision loss in your upper right quadrant, as you can see on the printout." He handed me the sheet.

"We need to perform some more in-depth research as to why this has come about, but I'll coordinate with Dr. Huizenga on that for you. I can't do anything more here in this office." I looked at my printed chart—the test results showed two black holes (one for each eye) where no pinprick of light could reach my brain—no life there. That spooked me. I quietly wondered if he had some ideas but didn't want to share them with me until he talked to Dr. Rob. (I found out later that I was right.) Despondent, I hiked back to Sam's.

She was there waiting with a turkey sandwich and lemonade.

"How'd it go?"

I sat down on the couch and finished half the sandwich as I described my doctors' visits. I told her about the biopsy Huizenga wanted to do and then said, "He thaid tad he wood tak to octor ahb . . ." I froze. *What the hell was that?!* Why was I slurring my speech? I looked at Sam in surprise, but her face was a stone mask. (I've come to learn that this is how she responds to trauma: she freezes and assesses.)

"Do . . . yhou . . . ear . . . dadh? Cahn . . . yhou . . . ear . . . mah . . . ords . . . shlurrinh?" To me, I sounded drunk. It was eerie. I knew what was happening to me, and I couldn't believe it.

"Yes, I hear that," she assured me. "I think we need to get you to the hospital. Let's go."

I stood up off the couch and nearly fell. I could barely walk. My adrenaline was giving me the shakes, even worse than during the car episode. For the first time in my life I had no control over my own body. Gizmoe, Sam's eight-pound Brussels Griffon dog, understood "crisis," and she beat us to the door, trying to slip past us into the hall.

"Caw–Dah–tah–Huith–en–ga," I said, trying with all my might to enunciate my words as my world collapsed. Sam pressed her cell phone as she helped me to her car, telling them we were headed to Cedars.

We were there in minutes. Sam parked near the ER and helped me out of the car. As we slowly walked across the parking lot, I looked up at the building we were about to enter—Cedars Sinai Hospital. How many times had I driven by this place without giving it a thought? Hospitals were for sick people. The flawless sky burned a silhouette of the looming building into my brain. Reality was too challenging. My world became just snapshots.

I saw my left arm. It was a creepy shade of blue. The fingers were purple. I saw Sam, supporting my weight and keeping me upright. I saw my feet walking on the pavement. I looked at the sky again and thought, *I'm gonna die today. Wow. I never thought it would end like this. I was going to live to ninety. I was going to have a big career in Hollywood. I was going to have kids.*

Suddenly, through all the craziness and nerves and panic, just before entering the building I hit a calm button. Yes, I was calm and ready to give in to it because I understood I had no choice in the matter.

Oh, God. This is so strange. I have so much left to do.

Sam waved at the triage nurse, who immediately fetched a tall doctor, a friend who Dr. Huizenga had called. They were expecting me. The nurse brought a wheelchair and I sat clumsily. *Ow.* With every movement, my brain sloshed around in my skull. I fought to organize the blurry pictures. I let the nurse position my feet on the rests and wheel me to a room in the ER. I struggled with the comprehension that this was all beyond me now. I was dying, and it was only a matter of—it didn't matter, actually.

Just make it go fast, please.

"Kevin. Are you taking any steroids?" the nurse asked.

I looked at her. The question actually angered me. "No," was all I could muster.

Thoughts swarmed my head, like when a cartoon character gets bonked: little tweeting birds and number signs and exclamation points. So much was happening. Sam and the nurse helped me onto the bed as I tried to explain about the slurred words and the lump in my shoulder. My speech was sounding more normal. To my confused brain, though, it didn't seem to concern them much either way. I wondered why they kept asking questions, why they couldn't see that I was dying.

"How long have you been lifting weights? Have you taken anything else? Drugs? Do you drink alcohol? Do you take anything to help you bulk up? Steroids? How about any supplements?"

"No," I repeated. I abhorred drugs of any kind.

"He doesn't even drink coffee," Sam interjected.

The doc was on top of things, ordering a barrage of exams.

For the final test in the ER cubicle, they wanted another echocardiogram. In order to get the best possible picture of my heart, this one required me to "swallow" the camera.

"Ma'am?" The nurse was talking to Sam. "We're going to have to ask you to leave the room now."

PRINCE CHARMING

Sam Sorbo

As a working actress in Los Angeles, my career had taken me many places, but New Zealand was a new, exotic destination to add to my list. I sat in business class on flight 821 from LAX to Auckland, listening to the pilot explain that our flight was canceled due to volcanic activity. Mt. Ruepehu, on the North Island, is the largest active volcano in New Zealand—and one of the world's most lively. The delay would be at least twenty-four hours, depending on the mountain.

The next day, with the cooperation of the volcano, I arrived in New Zealand only twenty-four hours late. Being delayed by a day caused me to miss the standard cast read-through, during which all the actors gather around a large conference table and read aloud their parts in the script. I was the guest star on the episode, playing Princess Kirin, and the director understandably required a meeting between the show's star and me before filming.

First, I had a costume fitting: lots of push-up bras built into the outfits to ensure that the show lived up to its nickname, "Baywatch, B.C." I never knew I could look so busty! Then I walked to the read-through, which was at a small apartment building not far from the hotel. I rang the bell and Charlie, the director, introduced himself cheerfully and waved me in. He was happy, no doubt, at not having to recast a heavy, pivotal role with a local actress the day before shooting.

I, however, was still a little worried. What was the star of the number-one show in the world going to be like in person? He was good looking. He was successful. I had done my time with less accomplished actors who were so full of themselves they wouldn't come out of their trailers when asked, preferring to make the crew wait. The most recent one of them in particular had been a mean, rude brute of a guy. Here I was supposed to have a love story with this Sorbo, and our first scene, the goodbye scene—a kissing scene—was scheduled for the following night! I knew I'd need to break the ice, and quickly. (The short funny phone call we shared the previous week hardly counted.)

Kevin Sorbo, fresh from the gym showers, lumbered into the director's cozy, rented apartment shortly after I arrived. The space immediately seemed much smaller to me.

I stood up to meet Kevin, and he said, "Hey, you're tall. That's good . . ."

I'm five-foot-ten. "Yes, I am!" I smiled and hugged him hello.

He awkwardly hugged me back, patting my shoulder in a brotherly fashion, saying, "Oh! Okay, we'll do the Hollywood thing . . . "

It was such an unexpected response; I was intrigued. Also, I should add, he had amazingly blue eyes. I stared into them a little too long.

"Okay, then, let's get to the script," Charlie broke in, distracting us from the odd, quiet tension in the room. We all sat down, and for the next hour we read through it aloud, with Charlie filling in for various parts. We finished up the evening discussing the characters and script elements, and Kevin offered me a ride home. I gratefully accepted, though it was only four blocks. I was exhausted, it was dark out, and I couldn't deny the electricity I felt between us.

The next day my call-time was 3 p.m. My first scene with Kevin would shoot at night—the end of a long week for him. I sat in the makeup chair as Annie transformed me into a princess. I had a long, flowing half-wig to augment my own hair. I wore fabulous gold-embroidered silken robes. I felt downright royal.

The star of the show popped his head in the door to welcome me to set and, apparently, to flirt. He was in costume and full of energy. "Wow," he said at first. Then, "I see you met Annie. Is she treating you okay?"

"Why do you ask? Don't I look good?" I wondered if he would know how to take a taunt.

Annie laughed. "That's right, girly. Kevin, uh, what are you saying, exactly?"

"No, nothing . . . You look very princess-like," he said. He looked surprised but undaunted.

I blushed. "And you look . . . uh, mythic," I said, stumbling. I was leery of charming, good-looking men.

"I'll take that as a compliment."

"Well, it figures you would."

"Oh, you're a tough one!" he parried.

"If you can't stand the heat, get out of the makeup trailer." We all laughed.

"She's a cheeky one, Kevin," Annie said as she fussed with my wig.

"I guess I'll see you on set, then, Princess."

"Just make sure you know your lines!" I teased, smiling at him. He was easy and adorable. Working with him was going to be fun, for sure.

Once he had gone, Annie, with the excitement of a fortune-teller predicting a lottery win, declared that he obviously was interested in me because he never flirted like that with the other costars.

The other costars! Ah, yes, they did send a beautiful actress down from the States for each new episode. I had met my share of superficial pretty-boy actors, and I had too much pragmatism running through my bones to mistake "interest" for anything other than shallow posturing.

I gathered my wits back under my wig and shrugged off Annie's postulating. It was time for me to be on set.

My "castle" consisted of an imposing courtyard door set into a fifty-foot-long wall of painted wood and faux stone. Through it would be the inner courtyard, but because this was a TV set, it was just scenery backing and dirt. I chose not to look at that side—no reason to ruin my regal fantasy.

My door faced out onto a bridge over a moat and a wilderness currently populated by an obscured production crew. The set lights limited my vision to my immediate surroundings. Fog, wafting up from the moat, gave the castle a magical quality. Acting like a princess in this setting would not be difficult, although this was the farewell moment, the end of a grand love story for my character—a life-and-death scene.

Kevin and I rehearsed our lines at the castle entrance, with Michael Hurst playing Iolaus. I stood opposite Kevin, in flats, feeling improbably petite and feminine. Kevin's brawny physique was the stuff of fairy tales, honestly—especially here, in a foreign country, in my castle—and getting caught up in the moment was easy.

The scene ended with our goodbye kiss. Kevin kept losing his place in the script, leaving me wondering about his level of professionalism. It was a simple script—ridiculously easy. Finally, he blurted out, laughing, "Michael, help me out here!"

Michael backed away, shaking his head and holding his hands up in front of him, "I'm not touching this one, buddy. You're on your own."

There was something odd going on. For the star of the show to forget a few straightforward lines certainly made no sense. I was suspicious that they were trying to trick me or something, but I couldn't quite figure out how—or why, even. Aside from that, Kevin was so charming and witty; my intense attraction to him was hijacking me.

Each time we came to the kiss, instead we would stop the scene and say it. "Right, then the kiss." At one point during our rehearsal he cheekily asked, "So, when we do the kiss, tongue, or no tongue?" He was joking of course, but as any good negotiator knows, once you name it out loud, it's on the table as an option.

They needed to work on the lighting, so George Lyle, the first assistant director, asked us to step down for a moment. Kevin, Michael, and I returned to the canvas director's chairs that the crew had lined up for us off set. After a few moments of idle chatter I wondered loudly if anyone had any breath mints. Immediately, the three hovering makeup artists dove into their kits to oblige me. I flippantly said, "Oh, no, not for me. For Kevin."

Oooh.

Kevin, four seats down, heard me (as I had intended). Luckily, he laughed. Sometimes people don't respond well to my convoluted sense of humor, but he obligingly accepted a mint. I relented and took one as well.

A minute or two passed quietly. Then Kevin proposed, with a glint in his eye, "Maybe we should see if these work."

I cracked up. He was audacious! Two could play at that game, however. Never one to back down from a challenge, I agreed. (After all, we'd have to kiss eventually, I rationalized.)

I watched him, first for his reaction, then in simple amazement. He was determined to see this through. His muscular arms lifted him lightly out of his chair. His trademark long hair brushed against his jaw in the evening breeze. Goosebumps popped on my skin. Approaching me, I saw the man to catch me when I fell. Kevin gently placed one large hand on either arm of my flimsy director's chair. He leaned in slowly, then paused, looked in my eyes, and smiled.

I smiled too.

The makeup artists, the other actors, the crew, and their noise all faded away. The magical castle, superfluous now, disappeared too.

We kissed, and sealed a deal.

SIDELINED

Sam Sorbo

I RELUCTANTLY TOOK A CHAIR outside the ER room where Kevin lay. The medical staff had explained to me that they would give Kevin some Valium and perhaps another sedative as well in order to make the experience of this particular examination as easy as possible, but that I should not stay in the room. They needed to stick a camera down Kevin's throat to photograph his heart from inside his ribcage.

I heard some commotion from inside, and then a nurse came out and glanced around the ER central station. She called out to a very tall male nurse, by far the biggest person in the room. She glanced at me, watching her. "Jim!" she shouted again, trying to sound more casual. "Come give us a hand in here, please." I inferred from this that Kevin did not want that camera down his throat. He was a very big guy who, when it came to brute strength, usually got his way. Five of them were needed to hold him down.

After the procedure a nurse invited me back into his room. "Just keep him calm and don't let him pull out his IV. The sedative will wear off in a little while."

He was groggy but awake. Suddenly, he sat up, saying, "I have to get to the game." He scooted down the bed a bit, preparing to slip off, oblivious to his surroundings.

I grabbed him and said, "No, no! The game can wait. You stay right here."

He was determined. Quickly, I moved around behind him, hung one hand over his right shoulder, and wrapped my other arm around his waist. If he wanted to get off the bed, he would have to carry me too. Luckily, that proved too much of a challenge and he relented, falling back on the bed and then passing out.

Eventually, the doctor came back in the room with Dr. Huizenga and told me that Kevin's heart was fine. They wanted to do an MRI and maybe a CT scan as well.

It seemed like we waited forever for the MRI, but we got it done the same day.

We were also assigned a hospital liaison for Kevin who asked if he wanted to be checked in under a pseudonym. That seemed like a good idea, although at this point, we had no clue how serious things were.

Without any specific information to the contrary, I was in denial that this was a big deal. I had known Kevin for just over a year. We were engaged, and because of our work schedules, the time we had spent together was intense and dedicated. I knew him very well. He was the fittest, healthiest, and most active person I had ever met. He was incredible, overly capable, and simply unstoppable. I just assumed we would fix this weird health crisis and then life would return to normal. I admit I bought into the whole Hercules thing, hook, line, and sinker.

I was not the only one. While we were wheeling Kevin on his gurney to the MRI, no fewer than five individuals asked him for an autograph. The oddest thing, though, was that they expected Kevin to supply the pen.

STRANGE

Even on a good day an MRI is a torture device. They asked if I wanted earplugs. What I really wanted was for someone to take my brain, wring it out, clear out the humming, buzzing, throbbing, cobwebby stuff, and make it all go away. Earplugs being the only option, however, I accepted them. They had me lie flat on my back on a table, told me not to move, and then slid me into the long, narrow, white tube. I was completely claustrophobic. I tried closing my eyes, but it's like going across a tightrope: Once you look down, the depth of your potential fall is all your mind can see. Then there is the deafening pounding of the machine as it works: relentless clicking, ticking, and thumping. But because I felt awful anyway, I became fully committed to any method that might find a solution to my problem.

The brain MRI was normal, but the shoulder MRI showed this:

1. 2 cm supraclavicular mass most likely representing a lymph node.
2. Small node approximately ¾ of a cm just adjacent to it.
3. It does not appear to be compressing the vascular structures that appears [*sic*] to be superior to it.

4. No disruption of the tissue planes identified.

5. There is no evidence for abscess or other inflammation.

Translation: It's a lymph node with another smaller one next to it, neither of which are affecting blood circulation. Further translation: *Probably cancer—but not a brain tumor.*

They did not tell us they suspected cancer. They only said they needed more tests on the funny lump on my shoulder.

I was admitted to a hospital room and promised more tests in the morning. I was exhausted yet completely wired. My head was spinning, that generator hummed in the back, and everything was still kind of watery and out of focus. The blind spot in my vision messed with me a lot, and Huizenga's evening assurances of being on track to finding the problem only seemed to emphasize the fact that no one knew what was wrong with me.

I thought about my parents. I was sure they would want to know, but we had not phoned them yet, deciding that, with no facts, worrying them would do no good. Now it was too late to call, anyway. Sam slept on the couch and I spent the night horizontal at least, but the dread that shrouded me when I had first entered the hospital lingered, frustrating any hope for sleep. I wanted to know what was wrong, but then again, I didn't.

Late the next morning they brought me down to the Doppler lab to run a test on my left arm. The Doppler maps internal tissues by using sound waves, kind of like how boats use sonar to see the bottom of the ocean.

The young technician, Julie, was proficient and pleasant. She methodically swept the wand over my arm and we watched the results feed out of her machine: red on white paper. Nothing noteworthy, unfortunately. The mundane results seemed to disappoint her a little.

I had my own reasons to be frustrated. With one more inconclusive examination, we seemed to be no steps closer to finding out what was causing my intense symptoms.

Then Julie said, "Since I'm here, I'm just going to look at the other side of your wrist. They don't ask for it on the req, but I figure, we may as well."

I shrugged. "Why not?" Where else was I to go?

The next thing she said is burned in my memory: "That's strange."

"What?" I demanded.

"I can't find a pulse, and you should have one over here . . . but you don't." She was massaging my lower forearm and wrist with the sensor, searching for some feedback.

No pulse meant no blood flow.

They rushed these results to my doctors. "Mr. Sorbo, you have severe disruption of blood flow in your lower arm. Two main arteries feed the hand, and one of yours is completely occluded. We are scheduling you for an emergency arteriogram, and we suspect that the lump on your shoulder is actually an aneurysm. We need to see inside there." *Of course. Do what you have to do, but let's do it now!* I wanted to scream. I nodded my head instead.

Mapping the blood paths in my left arm required inserting a tube into the large artery in my groin and then threading it up my torso, through my beating heart, and finally into my shoulder. Through it they injected some horrible, stinging dye into the area, x-raying the dye as it traveled with the blood in my system. The pain was intense. The added fluid swelled inside my arm, making it feel like a balloon. It was all I could do to remain still on the table. The entire procedure consisted of several similar tests, repositioning and replacing the catheters, and redirecting new shots of dye.

They wheeled me into the ICU for recovery. "Kevin, the lump in your shoulder is a large aneurysm that has been throwing clots for quite a while. You have a lot of blockages all the way down your arm, which explains your symptoms of cold fingers, tingling, and numbness that have been going on for months. There is no blood flow in much of your lower arm."

But now, at least, my doctors had a plan.

It was not an *ideal* plan.

It was more like a "Plan C."

"We've thinned your blood with powerful anticoagulants, and in the angio tube, we are pumping Urokinase straight into your arm and hand. It's a strong clot-busting drug. Now we have to wait to see if the drugs will do their job. We should see the results fairly quickly. We are doing our utmost to save your arm."

They crossed their fingers that the meds would clear out the clots and allow blood to flow. They hoped it would come in time. It was the best they could offer.

But there was a catch. While I lay horizontal, looking up at him, Dr. Huizenga continued, "Kevin, listen to me because this is serious. Basically, you are a drug-induced hemophiliac right now, and you have a sizeable hole in your groin. You may not move at all. You may not sit up or even move your legs around. If the hole in your groin tears or you accidentally injure yourself, we will have a very hard time stopping the blood flow."

In short, no walking, no sitting, no stretching, and no crapping (which meant no eating). Of course, I had a catheter. Of course, I needed a workout. Of course, I was starving. I was accustomed to eating six to seven times a day, and I had only picked at the hospital's turkey and mashed potatoes the night before. Anxiety could repress my appetite for only so long before my body began demanding food, as it was now.

I swallowed. My mouth was dry. "For how long?"

"We'll need to take it day by day. We'll do more tests in the morning to see how the drugs are performing. With luck, you'll be off it sooner rather than later. But Kevin, you have a lot of blockages in your arm. We are doing all we can to save it. You need to be patient and let the drugs do their work."

My mind was a list of questions. "Okay, but what about when my speech slurred? Where does that fit in here?"

"It does sound like you suffered a couple of ministrokes, Kevin, but they didn't show up on the MRI. The one in your speech center passed, so we can hope that the vision one will too—there's no way to tell except time. We'll be watching for any further issues in your head as well, going forward, but for now, we are dealing with the aneurysm and your arm."

I wished that reassured me, but my head was sending another message.

Regardless, my immediate instructions were clear: *Don't move.*

The idea of checking in under a pseudonym turned out to be good foresight. I was not ready for the press to blast my illness to the world. However, now that I had a grasp of what I was up against, I had to tell my producers. I was supposed to be in Atlanta filming *Black Dog*, a movie about a trucker who is haunted by his traumatic past. The production staff of this film called the insurance company and suspended all production matters until further notice. (Because of the movie, *Hercules* wasn't scheduled to start up again for almost another three months.)

I was due on Terry Bradshaw's new talk show on the eighth. We canceled, and because of that, my health condition became public. Universal Studios' executives, my agent, and my manager decided it would be prudent to keep the details confidential for the time being. My TV character was invincible, so we couldn't have me seem too vulnerable. I am naturally a private individual, so that worked for me.

CNN ran my hospitalization on their ticker tape, and *Entertainment Tonight*, *Extra*, and many other news sources also broadcast my health trouble. *Army Archerd* published an announcement of my aneurysm and hospitalization at Cedars on September 9. None of them knew the extent of my injuries or the severity of the issue. We let the publicist spin something about it being fully treatable.

Even I bought that story. Almost.

ICE CREAM

Sam is talking to me. God, she is a beautiful girl—long and lean, joyful and creative. Her mind moves quickly, finding humor easily and offering graceful challenges too. I wish I could just take her hand and walk out of this room, but I am fixated in the bed—by the tubes, by the machines, by my panic.

She is saying something about a TV commercial, ice cream, and New York. Man, it's hard to concentrate. My head just does not want to join the party. After two days on my back, unable to move or even stretch, I have reached my limit. Angry thoughts crowd my throbbing brain.

She asks if she should turn it down—her commercial job in New York.

Really? Is she really asking that?

No . . . but yes, in fact.

She is clearly elated about the job: national network. Those are the good ones to book, for sure.

"Ice cream, my favorite thing in the world!" she beams.

I smile at her, though I'm not sure it masks my scowl. I am irritated and frustrated. Of course, the three-day commercial shoot in New York City would be great. But I am stuck, as my sweat seals my discomfort. Twenty-four hours on my back already, and counting. *Doesn't she understand—my life is over and I don't give a crap about ice cream! I can't even have food!*

I met Sam at a time when I had finally given up on ever finding someone to share my life with. She appeared with her charming humor and
irresistible beauty. I was immediately smitten. Then I got a load of her
intelligence and I thought, here was the woman I was looking for, not
simply attracted to. Okay, maybe it wasn't *that* specific, but honestly, the
weekend after we first met, I was strangely fantasizing about starter
homes with swing sets. Trust me, that's not my usual fantasy.

I have always been an impatient man. Sam's stint in New Zealand
would be less than two weeks total. There was no time to waste. On our
third day of shooting (five days after we first met) I asked her point
blank, "How are we going to make this work?"

"Make what work?" she said, innocently.

I laughed. *As if she didn't know!* I mean, from that first kiss . . . "*This.*" I
indicated with my hands the immense attraction between us. "What are
we going to do about the water hazard?"

She looked at me skeptically. Obviously, my golf references were completely lost on her. (Even that I could forgive!)

"You know. The Pacific Ocean," I explained.

She could move each eyebrow independently, and was looking at me
with one up and one down, like *I* was the crazy one! Could she be that
dense? Didn't she understand that this connection we had was perma-
nent and undeniable? Apparently, yes, because she answered me in
measured tones: "I don't date actors. I don't date long distance. And I
don't date guys with long hair . . ."

Well, I changed all that for her, just like she redefined my intentions. I
broke all of her rules, but now, lying prostrate in a hospital bed, I wonder
if she has another rule about dating basket cases, if that's a rule I should
even attempt to break. I don't have my brain, my body is failing me, and
my career is uncertain. Sam is all I have left of my dream life.

There was never an opportunity for her to witness my weakness. What
weakness? I had none that I admitted, except that I'm a romantic—but
chicks dig that, I know it, so it doesn't really count.

Now I'm lying on a hospital bed in the ICU. I feel like Sam can look
through me; I must be worthless in her eyes, a dead weight. She should

turn and walk, go shoot the commercial, never look back. Why should she stay?

But she is the only reason I am rousing my energies each day. Why else? For my manager's visits? My agent? My lawyer? They're not coming back. They made the obligatory visits at first, but no one seems to understand what I'm going through. Except for Sam. My parents would make the trip, but I don't want to alarm them or impose on them like that. My brothers and sister, well, they have their own lives. New Zealand was halfway round the world. We have grown apart, much to my disappointment. I don't really have any close friends in LA anymore, either. Living an ocean away makes sustaining friendships difficult.

I wish I could tell Sam to go do her thing, that I'll be here waiting when she gets back. But let's face facts: Pathetic is the new me. My tattered ego cannot overcome the loneliness the tubes and the machines impose, nor the fear of what's happened inside my brain, the elephant we have yet to name. So I decide I am not above begging. I don't really care how she feels about me, as long as she stays.

"Congratulations on the job offer. Ice Cream. Awesome. When does it shoot, again?"

"I'd have to leave tomorrow," she says sweetly, honey in dirt.

No, Sam. Don't go to New York, not even for two days, not even for a moment. I need you here. I need you, please.

Tears are welling on her lower eyelids. She pretends it's just normal; she cried often enough before I got sick—tears of joy for her birthday earrings, tears of love when I proposed. But I can tell that these come from concern, even pity. She has never seen me so vulnerable. Hell, I've never seen me so vulnerable. This sucks.

"It would be great if you stayed here," I admit, wishing I had something, anything, to offer her.

"Of course," she says. "No problem." *She understands.* She steps outside to call her agent and turn it down.

I am so relieved, I even smile.

Sam returns, seeming calm and matter-of-fact. I wish I could be. I vividly remember the voice of warning in my ear, and now I understand that I messed up, big time, by not heeding its message.

"Don't let him crack your neck."

That voice. I hear it again, like a bad children's song that ceaselessly haunts my thoughts. I want to change the tune. I long to hear the soft, steady timbre of that voice again, telling me something good, something of comfort. But it's the same old song.

I gather a deep breath and then let it out slowly so Sam won't notice how f-ing terrified I really am.

TERRIFIED

Sam Sorbo

AFTER HIS FIRST NIGHT in the ICU the doctors ordered a second angiogram to see how the clots were responding to treatment. They had just wheeled him back from the operating room. A male nurse was reorganizing the machines around him and double-checking their settings.

I watched him on the bed. He was despondent. "Hey, your brother Tom called last night. And your parents. I told them a trip out here was unnecessary, but they can't wait to talk to you. We'll figure this all out and then you'll get out of here and we'll be laughing about this, soon. How did it go in there this time?" I tried to be upbeat, certain this entire ordeal was only a minor setback. He would be just fine.

During Kevin's time in the hospital with no access to a phone, the job of calling his family and friends fell to me. I had reassured his parents it wasn't that serious. Besieged by decisions and out of an innate, knee-jerk reluctance to admit to them, or myself, the gravity of the situation, I asked them not to come. In hindsight, my response was regrettable.

I just refused to believe that anything could really touch him; to me, he was an amazing force of nature. My mind flashed back to when I discovered him practicing the fight choreography from our first episode together on the set in New Zealand. The weather was chilly, and he wore his royal blue fleece robe open over his costume. He was expert with the staff, his kicks were high and strong, and his spins made his long hair whip around his face. He was entirely focused on his moves until he was done and noticed me standing there. I, in contrast, was completely incompetent with fights. What I wouldn't have given for an ounce of his athleticism and grace.

"It kills when they pump the dye, or whatever, in my arm. I'm so ready to be done with this. And my head is just pounding." In spite of the pain, he looked strong and stoic. "It's really cold in here."

He started to tremble.

"It's okay, sweetie. I'll get you a blanket . . . "

Then the entire bed started shaking. Kevin shuddered violently without stopping. He looked at me, panicked. "Sam? Saaaam! Whaaaat's hahappepepenining?"

The nurse was still hovering as the bed wrenched on its locked wheels. Aside from my obvious concern about why he was seizing, I knew that a twitch in the wrong direction could tear something, and then the bleeding would be overwhelming.

The nurse must have been thinking along the same lines. "I need help in here!" he shouted, to nobody in particular. "We need to get this guy back into the OR or we're gonna lose him!" He pointed at me, "You need to leave, miss! You can't stay in here!" as another nurse came in.

I gasped and backed out of the room. I ran to the pay phones down the hall and dialed Dr. Huizenga's office. They put me through to him immediately. "He's convulsing and the nurse just said we may lose him! I don't know what to do! Please come down here!"

Then my dam broke, and I sobbed as he softly but firmly reassured me. "Sam, I'm sure they are doing everything they can. I will call my colleague to have him check in as well. Just sit tight. He is in excellent hands, and I will be there as soon as I can."

Blah blah blah . . . "Excellent hands?!" The nurse in there just scared the living daylights out of both of us, and I had no clue what they were doing to him now. What had gone wrong with the procedure? How were we going to fix this?

But what was I expecting? Dr. Huizenga couldn't just materialize out of thin air. He didn't have a magic wand to wave. My frustration closed around me like a fist. Determined to fix things for Kevin, I purposefully walked back into the ICU, recovering my optimism en route. We had caught this in time to save his arm (I hoped), and we would fix the rest of him as well, God willing.

What I discovered amazed me. Kevin was still in his room, calm and unmoving. There was someone in a white coat who introduced himself as a doctor.

"Kevin just had an adverse reaction to the procedure, but nothing a little Benadryl in his IV couldn't handle. He's stable now, and everything's fine." Then he left before I could even formulate a question.

I took Kevin's right hand, leaned my face over his, and stroked his cheek. He was pale. "You're okay now, Kevin. This will all be over soon. Don't you worry. I don't know what that was back there, but they fixed it and you're going to be fine." I fought to smile through my tears. I did not want him to see how afraid I was. I wanted him to be able to look at me and find solidity and strength.

In the back of my mind, though, I wondered what that episode was about. Benadryl? Really? Was this going to be the new normal? Seizures and emergencies?

It was like a shove from behind, and my paradigm shifted: day into night. The incredible tour de force I adored was an all-too-mortal man in serious jeopardy.

I heard a riddle once:

You are driving in a storm, and you pass a bus stop where three people wait:

1. An elderly woman who needs a hospital
2. An old friend who once saved your life
3. Your soul mate who you will never see again

Who do you pick up in your two-seater car? (This is a momentous decision, so consider it carefully.)

Since meeting Kevin over a year before, I had wrestled with the idea of splitting my life between two continents: marrying him and being with him in New Zealand while maintaining my career in Los Angeles. A half-season on Chicago Hope assured me of a promising future in acting. I had also been successful in my modeling career. My quandary was how my life would look—factoring in the long-distance thing, how I would divide my time and apportion my energy.

Then, like the first red rays of sunrise, the answer appeared. Facing the clear prospect of losing Kevin permanently forced me to acknowledge that he was more important to me than anything else. Being thrust in the position of decision maker also clarified that he needed me— more now than he ever would have before.

Solution? Simple. I just wanted him, first, last, and always. What good was the rest of it without him? No amount of ice cream, no Emmy or Oscar, nothing that I could buy with the gobs of money I might earn with professional success would ever measure up to him in my heart. He was what I had been waiting for. I had known it within a week of meeting him, even while the distractions of career and life duped me into assigning everything else some equivalent value. Now I saw that none of the rest mattered without him in the mix.

Some may label my decision as a compromise. It was anything but. Once I finally saw it in black and white, life or death, not having to juggle all the balls was a relief. I craved spending time with Kevin, and he needed me too. I easily conceded all the rest.

The answer to the riddle is that you give your good friend the car to drive the old woman to the hospital while you stay with your true love through the storm.

You can't have it all. You must choose to find happiness—and then commit to it.

So I gave all of myself to him, right then, in an ICU room in LA.

WHATEVER *YOU* THINK

"FOR ME, IT'S LIKE A WALK IN THE PARK!" Dr. Franklin Moser emphasizes with a disarming smile. "You have to understand, I do this in people's brains every day. The shoulder's so much easier. Plus, you've got the whole thing set up for my procedure right now. It's a—excuse me—*no-brainer*."

It has been forty-three hours of lying as still as possible—torture for my type-A personality. Yesterday morning they did another burning angiogram and still saw lots of clots, so they left everything as it was and sent me back to the ICU.

This morning, more flames down my arm, more dye. I only feel worse each day, but I am told I am making progress.

The intense morning sun slashes through the blinds at Dr. Moser, who stands by my bed talking energetically. He is maybe a few years older than I am, with thinning hair—a neuroradiologist and a very smart guy. He is dedicated and enthusiastic about his specialty. Sam and Huizenga listen intently, and I try to focus on his words.

"This is not the conventional treatment for a shoulder aneurysm, but it's less invasive. I can use the angiogram tube that is already in place to insert a platinum coil, or coils, into the aneurysm. The blood should then clot around the coils and adhere to the walls of the aneurysm, effectively neutralizing it. Eventually, within several weeks, the aneurysm will be side-lined, 'clotted off.' The coil-clots should form a new arterial wall that will allow blood to flow as normal through the area."

They talk across me almost like I am not there, yet then they address me as if I can participate in this big decision.

Yesterday we interviewed the best surgeon the hospital can offer, and he was confident he could cut out the aneurysm with minimal collateral damage (minimal being the operative word). Cutting into the shoulder, he clarified, necessarily exposed me to other risks. For instance, there is a critical breathing nerve that runs right through the area in question. If it is damaged during surgery—though it wouldn't be, he assured us—but just in the outside case that it might be . . . *I kind of like breathing*, I thought.

Moser finishes making his case and leaves us so we can deliberate.

"Typically, Kevin, you would be referred to surgery and that would be that," Dr. Huizenga says. "They don't treat aneurysms of the body like they do brain aneurysms, but I was thinking, why not? That's why I wanted to talk to Moser, because he's the best brain guy we have here. Now you've seen what he says, and the decision is yours."

Okay, I hear that part about deciding something, but in truth I couldn't follow the conversation up to then because of the blistering jackhammer in my brain. My back cries out to a deaf audience. I'm starving. Waah waah waah. I sound like such a crybaby, and I'm suddenly filled with adult-sized contempt for myself.

I know Dr. Huizenga has my best interests at heart, and I'm lucky Sam is here fighting for me, because I really have no clue what they were talking about. As they were weighing the pros and cons of each option, I was basically just nodding.

"Dealing with the aneurysm through the angio is much less invasive. Healing will be faster, and no scarring, right?" Sam used to volunteer in this hospital. She enjoys all the medical mumbo-jumbo.

"Right," Dr. Huizenga replies.

Sam looks at me. Perhaps she thinks I might have a question or some other important contribution to the discussion. I don't.

She continues, "If we try the embolization and it doesn't work, surgery is always an option, right?"

"Yes, of course," Dr. Huizenga answers.

"Kevin? What do you think?" Sam smiles at me, willing me to be happier in my situation.

Her will is no match for my aggravation.

What do *I* think?

Get me the hell out of here, actually. *This sucks!*

Frankly, I'm not convinced it even matters. I still feel like something is seriously wrong, like I am fading away, receding into some misty trap inside my brain, if only a little bit slower than I was when I first walked into the ER.

"Sure. If Dr. Rob says it's a good idea, I guess so . . ." I respond.

Sam strokes my lower leg. "Let's do it. There really isn't a downside, and Moser seems confident too. I think it'll be good." I wonder, *Is it possible for someone to be too optimistic?*

"Yes, I agree." Dr. Huizenga seems happy with the decision—confident.

"Yeah, good. Okay, so, when?" There is no concealing my impatience.

Huizenga looks down at my immobile form. He is not a demonstrative guy, having worked so long in professional football, where there are no babies. I must look really bad, because he places his hand gently on my good shoulder and pronounces, "Kevin, we've got to make sure we've done all we can to remove the clots before we can do any procedure to correct the aneurysm. Only one more day—that's the longest we'll risk shutting down the rest of you to try to save your arm."

That phrase sticks in my thoughts. Of course, loss of circulation means dying tissue, dead arm. I clench my fist. The bloated pain reassures me it is still there—for now.

SHOWTIME

I step out of the limo into a crowd of paparazzi—everyone smiling, jostling for a view, shouting at me.

"Kevin!"

"Mr. Sorbo, over here!" The blinding flashes are relentless and dizzying, but uplifting, too, glittering jewels on velvet.

They are here to see me, to photograph me and get my autograph, and I am dazzled and proud. I take a moment to look down at the dirty New York City sidewalk, and I smile to myself. I can barely believe it. Here I am, a small-town guy with a dream of making it in Hollywood, having just wrapped principal photography on a major studio picture, *Kull, The Conqueror,* which could position me as the next major action hero on the silver screen. I am about to promote my number-one-worldwide hit TV show on *Letterman.*

I hold my hand out for Sam and she steps into the glare with me. People are shoving, pushing my photo in front of me, holding out Sharpies for my autograph.

"Could you please sign this for me, Mr. Sorbo?"

"Kevin, I love your work, man. Here, please just sign this here?" I always stop to sign things for fans. I owe them a deep debt of gratitude.

"When's your movie coming out?"

"Hercules! Kevin! Hercules!"

"How about a picture with Sam? Kevin! Right here, please!" I wrap my arm around Sam's waist and squeeze, and we smile into the flashing lights.

The security guard at the back door of the Ed Sullivan Theater in New York, where they shoot *Letterman*, taps me gently on the back of my shoulder and politely offers, "Right this way, sir." I shake a few more out-reached hands and we walk inside, past a security desk, and down a bleak, narrow hallway. Up two flights of service stairs to another drab, florescent hall, we are shown into a small room that has my name on a piece of paper taped to the door.

My room has some cool stuff waiting for me, including a *Late Night* mug that I have to this day. My publicist, Peg, is there too. I grab a couple of grapes and a piece of cheddar and wait for the segment producer.

Jim knocks and opens the door. He is a small guy who looks like a teenager (he's probably more like twenty-five), and he projects a pur-poseful calm, which does absolutely nothing to conceal his anxiety. It is his responsibility to produce me as a guest for the live show, but of course, he really has no control over what I might say. It is that way for him with each guest he is assigned—poor guy. Consequently, Jim is a bit of a micromanager.

"I just want to go over the topics Dave's going to cover with you. First of all, it's an all-Kevin spectacular. Kevin Kline is the first guest, then you, and then Kevin Anderson. We've got every other Kevin known to man—all the staffers are going to be recognized! By the way, tonight is inter-national joke night, so if you have a good joke, that'd be great. Kline is going to do one in French, I think. No pressure, though." In rapid fire he goes over all the things we had discussed in the pre-interview, the phone conversation when they determine which of your stories merit repeat-ing for the host and audience.

I know from previous experience that Dave is quite comfortable rolling with the punches. He's an expert comedian who knows how to exploit even an unexpected or tense situation to get a laugh. I think all the prep work that Jim is doing is overkill, but I just go with it.

After he leaves Sam taps me on the shoulder. She flew into New York just to see me on my way back Down Under. "I've got the perfect joke for you!" she offers.

"I want to tell one that relates to New Zealand, though." We brainstorm for a minute and come up with a great solution. Honestly, I am surprised Jim doesn't come back to double-check on the joke.

Dave keeps the theater a little colder than the North Pole. I think this is so he doesn't fall asleep on the boring guests. Just kidding—Dave doesn't have boring guests! But the walk-in freezer of a stage certainly keeps me awake in spite of my jet lag.

After the introduction and a few questions about my show, Dave asks me if I have a joke to share for International Joke Night.

"For you, Dave, of course," I answer. "And since I shoot Hercules in New Zealand, I have a New Zealand joke for you. Knock-knock."

"Okay, who, uh, who's there?" Dave asks in his charming, guarded manner.

"The Interrupting Sheep."

"The Interrupting Sheep—"

"Baaahaahaahaa," I bleat, interrupting him.

The audience giggles. Dave deadpans for a beat, turning in to the camera, and we get a tremendous laugh. The audience is laughing, I am smiling, and Dave is loving it . . .

"Mr. Sorbo!" A grating voice breaks into my reverie. I wake into the stark white glare of the hospital that has been my home for six days. "I need to take your blood. Sorry to wake you."

A small, harried nurse in a baggy uniform is holding my left arm and tapping it to find the blood vessel. She scowls in concentration, then in consternation as I forcefully withdraw my arm. With my right hand, I point to the paper taped to the wall behind my left shoulder, which reads, "DO NOT TAKE BLOOD FROM LEFT ARM."

Wow. It seemed like only moments ago I was high on life, riding the most tremendous wave of joy and personal success. I had it all—the fame, the money, a gorgeous fiancée . . . right now I am supposed to be shooting my second feature film for Universal Studios. The opening of *Kull*, less than two weeks before, had been an extravaganza. I rode on a huge white stallion down Universal Studios City Walk, with hoards of fans lining the street. Now, suddenly, it's over.

Well, at least the fiancée is still there, grinning at me as she sashays into the room. "Hello, sleepyhead. They said you could eat, so I brought you spaghetti and meatballs from the Italian place across the street. Did you hear what Moser said? Aside from it being a success, I mean? Your arm should be fine—almost as good as new—because they got most of the big clots. He said it took thirty minutes of full pressure to staunch the blood flow when they removed the tube. Thirty minutes. That's some powerful drugs running through your system, Kevin. How are you feeling now, sweetheart?"

The nurse, a grumpy vampire in a Monet smock, has moved to the other side of the bed to find a vein in the correct arm. I smile wanly at Sam. "I'm starved, literally. Bring it on over here and let me at it." Sam snags the wheeled bed tray and lays it all out for me. "It smells fantastic. Thank you." Finally, something normal. I am moving in the right direction.

"You look so much better," she lies. "How is your head?"

"Man, it's killing me. There's this humming, and the dizziness is driving me nuts, but at least my head is off the pillow. I'm just happy to sit up. They told me to try to walk, like, to the bathroom or around the floor." I swallow some spaghetti. It feels solid in this liquid, unpredictable world.

"Before lunch I tried to get on my feet. I felt like I would topple over with every step. I'm so light-headed, Sam."

"Of course you are, honey. You haven't moved in a week, so your body is depleted."

I take another bite, then collapse back onto the bed. I confess, "My head just feels awful. There's like a fire raging back there. Here. Touch it. Can you feel it?"

Sam gives me her hand, and I place it at the base of my skull. "You're a little warm, but it feels fine."

"You can't feel the vibration? Really? You can't feel that burning?" I am so frustrated by this weird feeling of being out of the world. My reality is no longer everyone else's reality. "I just want to get out of here, Sam. I don't like this place. It's been too long already. Huizenga said I can't go home until I can walk easily. So I got up. I tried to walk to the bathroom.

But Sam, I . . ." I can barely control my voice. "My legs feel like someone else's legs. I have no strength left."

"You've been on your back for days now, without food. You can't run a marathon today, Kevin, as much as you might want to."

"No, I don't want to . . ."

She sits next to me on the bed. "You have been through a lot. Give it time, and don't be impatient, okay?"

"Yeah, I guess." She doesn't hear the vibration in my skull, can't appreciate how my head feels like a bowl of sludge. I look over at the nurse and see that her multihued top can now also boast another color: Sorbo Red, my blood. I decide not to embarrass her by mentioning it as she finishes up and leaves.

"And please be careful moving around, at least for the next few days, 'kay? If you do anything to open the wound, we will be seeing a lot of blood."

"You mean worse than this?" I say, holding up the blood-stained sheet.

Sam scowls at me. "I can tell you're feeling better. You're actually re-covering your sense of humor."

PART II
TITANIC

OUT OF THE FIRE

AFTER ANOTHER DAY in the hospital I was walking enough to earn my release. As I slowly entered Sam's condo, I saw the world though thick lenses—the couch and dog were very clear. My future, not so much.

Hercules brought down by an aneurysm. It seemed like a myth. How could I be severely ill? I was thirty-eight years old, in top shape. I had never even missed a day of school.

I wanted to reach out and touch everything, first, for balance, but also for the need to constantly reassure myself that what I was experiencing was real.

The day before, my doctor had sent me to the neurologist.

"So, we do suspect that you suffered a ministroke or two, which would account for the dizziness you are still experiencing as well as the vision loss. We aren't exactly sure why, though, as clots travel with the flow— they don't swim upstream. The aneurysm in your shoulder may be unrelated, but because we haven't documented any more in the last four days, we're going to release you and monitor your progress at a distance. The speech issue you reported has cleared up, and that's a good sign, and your MRI is clean, but I'd like to have you checked out by a neurologist here at the hospital as a final precaution."

Dr. Bookman's office was padded with books and traditional leather furniture. A conscientious, disciplined man, he had me stand and do the formal battery of tests:

"Flip your hand back and forth in your other palm."

"Stand on one foot and touch the tip of your nose with your out-stretched hand."

"Walk on an imaginary tightrope with one foot in front of the other."

Suffice it to say that I passed these with flying colors. I was a good athlete, used to doing choreographed fight scenes. Sure I was dizzy, and that generator buzz in the back of my head gave me no respite, but that didn't affect my hand-to-nose coordination. My balance was way off and my eyes felt sluggish, but Dr. Bookman was reassuring and optimistic when I mentioned how poorly I was feeling. He discouraged my fear that my head was really messed up.

Relieved to be out in the world again, my change in venue bolstered my resolve to heal myself. I was determined to return to my old gang-busters self, no matter what, and after my ordeal, a new project was just what I needed to focus on. I had four more days in LA before starting *Black Dog.*

On September 16 I arrived in Atlanta. A production assistant brought me to my apartment, a two-bedroom in a high-rise condo with a stately drive up and expansive *porte cochère.* I put down my bags and enjoyed the first silence of the day. From the large plate-glass windows, I could see forever; the entire city lay at my feet. I stepped back to explore my new digs. It was nicely furnished with plenty of space for my clothes, a desk for working, a fully stocked kitchen, and, I was told, a well-designed gym downstairs.

With the time difference, it still felt early, so rather than rest I rode the elevator down to the gym for a workout. Even the slight lift in the elevator taunted my low-grade nausea. I pedaled the recumbent bike for thirty-five minutes, just to get a sweat. It seemed to be a game of give and take: The bike workout made me feel better psychologically, but my head felt worse. My left arm throbbed.

The doctors had advised me to take it easy with the workouts for a bit, so I didn't attempt to lift with my arms. I sat on the leg press machine, put it at a light weight, and pushed. Easy. Back down and out one more time.

Then I felt a huge rush in my head—as if my brains were floating away. My eyesight went blotchy and my heart thumped hard in my chest. I barely managed to keep the weights from crashing down. I grabbed the holds on either side, as if they might prevent me from tumbling over. I sat, blinking, trying to will my brain into behaving. It was true—I had lost twenty pounds and had not been to the gym for over three weeks, a record for me, but this reaction to a little light leg work was horrifying.

I thought to myself, *What is wrong with you?*

Wait a minute . . . who was I kidding? The flight in from LA had knocked me on my ass—totally wiped me out. My head was exploding. I needed some rest.

Part of me wondered why I'd even come here.

You go to work; that's what you do, I reminded myself.

Retreating to my apartment, I took a long, hot shower and didn't feel much better. In fact, I was even more depressed. I had an awful feeling that they had missed something at the hospital. What if the cause of the blood clots in my brain were unrelated to my aneurysm, as some of the doctors believed? What if I also had a brain aneurysm? What if bad things happen in threes?

Fuck this. They told me they had fixed it.

I closed my eyes and tried, unsuccessfully, not to think.

Day one on *Black Dog*: rehearsals and a costume fitting—a short day. When I arrived at the production offices the producer (and my friend), Raffaella De Laurentiis, greeted me with a smile. We kissed cheeks, as they do in Italy, and she said, "Kay-vin. You are feeling okay again, yes?"

"Yeah, thanks. Ready to get to work!" I answered cheerfully. I met the director and all the actors, including Meat Loaf and Randy Travis, which was very cool. We read through the script, grabbed lunch, and then a production assistant brought me over to a large, empty parking lot to take some driving lessons on an eighteen-wheeler. The focus required to handle the big rig preoccupied me enough to keep my head problems at bay, and that night I dropped on the bed and slept a lot. Finally.

The next few days I had more rehearsals along with makeup and wardrobe tests, when they check how everything plays for the camera and make last-minute adjustments. Trucker clothes are pretty easy, and makeup was a snap too, so we finished quickly and then the rest of the day was mine. Being back in the saddle again felt good, but in spite of my enthusiasm there was a persistent gray pall over everything. I still didn't feel like the old me. I had a deep dread that I was not healthy, and my fear was gradually eclipsing the part of me that insisted everything was terrific, overshadowing any faith I had in my doctors.

Throughout the first day of shooting the molten drone in my head had intensified. I struggled to stay focused, but somehow I managed to keep it all together. I had a 7:00 A.M. call and wrapped at 6:12 P.M., heading directly home. It felt like the hardest I had ever worked in my life, though Lord knows I had days on *Hercules* that were much longer and physically tougher. That night, I just collapsed in bed.

Awake at 4:15 A.M. I did my new routine systems' check while lying in bed. Still dizzy? Check. Head? Set to low, but still humming. Nothing had changed, there. I stretched my arm, flexed my fingers, and then balled them into a fist. Still tingly and painful, but manageable, I reasoned.

After some Advil and cardio, I showered and ate. By the time Todd, my driver, arrived, I was waiting for him in the lobby.

I checked in for hair and makeup, feeling pretty upbeat. The makeup artist was a woman in her mid-forties with short red hair and a quick smile. She spoke with a slight drawl and I found out she was from Texas, so we chatted about Dallas, where I had spent some time after college. I went to my camper, got dressed, and they called me to set.

The Atlanta autumn crisped the air around us on the cold asphalt of our parking-lot set. I rubbed my hands together in the early morning chill. Filming a movie is a lot slower than filming television. We blocked the scene, shot the master (a wide shot), and I went back to my trailer to wait for the crew to adjust the lights for the close-ups.

I lay down inside the camper. I could feel my adrenaline buzz fighting with the dizziness that wouldn't abate. I tried to ignore it. For distraction, I brought my 7-iron over to show Kevin Hooks, our director and an avid golfer like me. We made small talk about my club and my new grips.

Suddenly, the world caved in—much worse than at the gym the other night. My head began churning on overdrive, like marbles in a blender. I carefully excused myself from Kevin and started back toward my camper. This time, I felt like there were needles being jammed into me from all angles. I was shivering, nauseated, and I felt like crawling, like scratching all my skin off. I needed to be anywhere but inside me.

Breathless, I quietly told an assistant director, and he called for the set medic, Greg, who found me pacing in my trailer.

"Thanks for coming," I said, laboring for words.

"Sure. What's going on?"

"I'm not sure what's happening." My head was ablaze. "I've got shakes and chills, and I keep getting these head rushes. I'm light-headed, really dizzy." Maybe my body was finally giving up.

The cast and crew were depending on me. I felt guilty to be succumbing to this, whatever this was. I know it sounds stupid, but I felt so useless and weak—certainly not like Hercules. How could this be happening? To *me?*

Greg was calm and efficient, "Sit down here, Kevin, so I can take a look at you." He examined my hands and asked me, "Do you have any chest pain or difficulty breathing?" I shook my head. My heart was rhythmless and my blind spot was growing, turning things black. But all I said was, "No . . . not that."

While he took off the blood pressure cuff, I called Dr. Huizenga in LA, who told me to wrap myself in a blanket and walk. I did as directed, but the shivering did not go away. My sense of dread intensified, like a knife being sharpened, and I could focus on nothing else. I dialed the number of a local physician next, and he told me to get to the hospital.

Greg wasn't taking any chances, either. He called for an ambulance. Raffaella was on set, got the news over the walkie-talkie, and made a beeline over to me. I could see the concern in her face, reflecting back into my paranoid haze.

I knew it was too good to be true.

SECOND TIME AROUND

IN MY TWENTIES, five years before *Hercules*, I dated a great girl named Beth, whose father was a big booster for the USC Trojans football team. On our first date I met, among others, Ronnie Lott, Charles White, Marcus Allen, and even Lynn Swann. These guys were my football heroes growing up as a jock in little old Mound, Minnesota. It was all a bit surreal for me.

As that sports-driven kid, I used to think my father, Lynn, had a really wussy name. (Not to be mean to my Dad, but . . .) Then along came All-Pro wide receiver Lynn Swann, who played NFL football for the Super Bowl champs of the '70s, the Pittsburgh Steelers. He was a superstar, with his four rings, and suddenly my dad's name was actually pretty cool.

Mr. Swann laughed when I told him that story, and we quickly became friends.

Lynn had a motorboat that we took out to Lake Mead occasionally for camping and water skiing. One summer weekend we were out on a boating trip with our girlfriends. That Saturday night around 3 A.M., while we were camped out on the beach sleeping, a boat pulled up about a hundred yards off the shore, shone two large floodlights on our tents, and started shooting at us. For real. With bullets. Nothing like the sound of a gunshot to wake you up.

It was petrifying. We were completely unarmed; we didn't even have cell phones because at that time they were still massive hunks of junk no one carried around with them.

We heard the guys on the boat laughing as they fired shot after shot. Drunk target practice. Lynn, the girls, and I took cover behind some rocks and tried to figure out how to make an escape. We had no idea how far our assailants were prepared to take the attack, but eventually they got tired of their game and drove off.

In the morning we filed a police report, but the bright floodlights had prevented us from getting even a description of their boat. There was nothing more to do. We set out to cruise the lake.

Lynn's boat had two anchors, each about thirty pounds of metal, shaped like two large spikes with a third prong pointed ninety degrees to the first two. He had dropped both anchors the night before to keep the boat in position at our cove, but as we set off that morning, probably because of all the madness, he forgot to weigh the back anchor.

We must have dragged it for several hundred yards, picking up speed as we went. I was sitting in front, next to Lynn, who was driving, but I turned to his girlfriend at the back of the boat and suggested we exchange seats. I took her place, sitting up on the back ledge of the boat with my feet on the rear seat, feeling the cool breeze and enjoying the beautiful desert sun on my face. Behind me, at the end of a long nylon rope, the anchor dragged along silently through the water.

About a minute after I sat down that anchor came flying up through the air like a torpedo. Its rope was like a slingshot, pulled taut by the water. When the anchor skipped above the surface it careened forward and slammed me. It hit me square on my back, catapulting me down to the floor between the forward seats and knocking me out.

I came to, coughing up blood, and I didn't even know why. Luckily, there were two doctors on a boat nearby who witnessed the event. They rushed over and checked me out. The blood I was spitting was from my teeth biting into my tongue from the force of the hit. It turned out my back muscle mass had prevented any disastrous internal injury, and the doctors remarked how lucky I was to be broadsided by the three-pronged anchor rather than impaled. I was also fortunate it hadn't hit my skull. I had egregious bruises up and down my spine for weeks, but amazingly, I was fine.

It is astonishing how fragile we are as well as how strong, but some guardian angels kept me safe from screaming bullets and flying anchors on that weekend at Lake Mead. I thought of that time more than once during my battle with this new unseen enemy, wondering if I might have already used up all my blessings.

"Mr. Sorbo, could I have your autograph?"

Traveling by ambulance is not as much fun as you might think when you are convinced you are dying. The blanket over me felt like a sheet of ice. I shivered uncontrollably. Memories of incongruent events flurried like a snowstorm. The siren blared, adding a panicked soundtrack.

Suddenly, the emergency medic in the ambulance had a touch of remorse. "When you're feeling better, I mean," he added.

There would be more requests as the day progressed, and I refused them all. People completely ignored my condition and the setting. Then again, I'm told I didn't look as bad as I felt, so maybe they thought I was in for a sprained ankle. Either way, at the time their feelings were the least of my concerns.

My shaking, I know now, was an adrenalin overload—my body fighting for survival. At the time it just felt like overwhelming terror, and all I could think was, *Shit, I'm dying. Shit. Shit. Shit. I'm dying, damn it! Why can't this leave me alone?*

The paramedics gave me something to calm my shivering, but it did nothing for my paranoia. By the time we entered the hospital emergency room, pessimism and fear reigned. I could not view the talented medical staff as anything but the last people I would see on earth.

Where was the poetry in that? I thought of my father, a farmer's son. He was a public school teacher who struggled and scrimped to give the five of us kids a better life. He loved, disciplined, and shaped me, and I owed him so much. This wasn't the way to leave him. And my mother, Ardis, who I adored. I thought of her bad back, the nineteen back surgeries she had over the past forty-five years and all her pain. I remembered as a kid overhearing them the last Friday of each month, budgeting the family finances at the kitchen table, trying to find a few cents here to cover a bill over there. When I was fifteen I promised to buy my mother a house. She smiled and said she just wanted me to be happy. Dying before her was not part of that.

I pictured Sam, the love of my life, the woman who changed me from a bachelor into an engaged man. I wished her exasperating optimism was here next to me now, assuring me it would all work out okay. I wanted to marry her, have kids with her, grow old with her by my side, but those images were fading away. I wanted to at least have the chance to tell her, "I told you so," and "I love you." I thought, with an odd twinge of jealousy, about the man she might find in my absence. *Asshole.*

My morbid, sarcastic thoughts, unleashed by the adrenalin, drowned out any hopefulness or confidence the technicians in the ambulance or the ER might have inspired. A nondescript nurse wheeled me in for another MRI. I was given earplugs. The spongy buds seemed to trap my reflections, which pinged around inside my brain as the jackhammer of the MRI pounded outside.

A battle waged, and, being the field, I was losing.

REVELATIONS

THE DOCTOR ENTERED my hospital room quietly. He took a moment, looking down at my chart. "Kevin, I got the new MRI results, and it does show three distinct strokes in your brain." He sounded mildly apologetic, like a cashier who gives you the wrong change.

"Since I got out of Cedars?" I was floored.

He shook his head. "No, no. Typically, strokes take at least three days to show up on the MRI scan. So, no, you probably suffered the strokes that you initially reported, but they weren't discernable on the first MRI. You aren't really at risk for more as long as the cause has been taken care of, which they determined was the aneurysm."

Sam, who had flown in the day before, jumped into the discussion. "But the doctors in LA told us that if it was a stroke, it was so small it wasn't visible on the MRI."

"Well, they couldn't have known from an MRI taken so quickly after the event. Typically it takes about three days for any damage to appear on the films."

"So they sent him out here without knowing the extent of the injuries? How . . . how could they do that?" Sam's voice cracked and her face was flushed. "What does your MRI show? He had *three* strokes?"

"Yes. Basically, exactly what Kevin told me, based on his symptoms. His balance center was affected in two areas, it appears, along with his sight. I'm pretty sure you didn't suffer another stroke yesterday because everything you described is consistent with a very pronounced panic attack, not a stroke. It was your body's way of telling you that you need to rest." He spoke carefully but quickly, laying it on the line. "You had three strokes, Kevin. Three. This is not a head cold. Any normal person would need months of rest and rehab. You are very lucky to be walking around. They could have left you far worse off, including dead." He paused for the weight of the statement to sink in. He continued, "Is there anything you want to ask me?"

"So, the dizziness and aching head and stuff—that's all because of strokes?"

"I would have to say yes."

"How quickly do you think it will go away?"

"Everyone is different, every brain unique. You're a relatively young man, Kevin, so your prognosis is much better than, say, a seventy-year-old. But, for instance, your vision might get better or it might not. Vision is one of the more stubborn parts of the brain in healing, although often the brain learns to adjust."

"Are you saying, 'No more movie'?" Sam, a bottom-line kind of woman, searched for clarity.

"Well, as a neurologist, it isn't my job to say." He turned back to me, gathering his thoughts. "Kevin, your brain is hurt. At some point it gives up, like it did yesterday. I cannot say how it will go from here. Only you can decide if you're well enough to continue working right now. I can prescribe some things to help you cope." He broke out the silver lining. "The good news is that this isn't a new medical issue."

The room was silent. Not a *new* medical issue? It hardly mattered, if it would put me back in the hospital every few weeks. I just kept thinking, *I hate drugs. I'm strong. I don't need a crutch.*

Clearly, I was in bad shape and needed to heal. But my neurologist, sending me back to work as if nothing had happened, leading me to believe—what, exactly? I had three bullets in my brain. He made it seem like they were so tiny, so insignificant. I wondered at his outwardly blithe approach, especially now that I was experiencing just how disruptive they could be. Perhaps he couldn't have known.

We would not discover until years later that, from the vision test, Huizinga and Castor suspected the first stroke immediately. After Sam witnessed my words slurring, they became even more concerned. Once they ruled out a heart valve problem, there were only two other obvious explanations: a brain tumor or some other form of cancer, especially in light of the large mass on my shoulder. Either way, they were very quiet about their suspicions at that time, probably to keep us both calm. Then, when the aneurysm was diagnosed, all their original hypotheses faded. Meanwhile, the strokes had seemed to stop, and the first MRI didn't show strokes, so the case was closed—at least until it resurfaced.

Although I had probably not suffered another stroke this time, I was still being confronted with the hard truth that I had definite and possibly irreversible brain damage. My fragile confidence in my doctors was shattered. My speech had healed right away, but the rest of the damage still lingered, and now I knew why. My reality was changing again, and I could do nothing to stop it.

"If it's any consolation, your case is fascinating. I did a little research on this kind of manipulation causing blood clots to swim upstream. There is a lot of controversy surrounding the chiropractic adjustments of the neck."

"Half the doctors we saw out west didn't believe the strokes had any-thing to do with the chiropractic," Sam offered.

"Yes, I'm not surprised. I'm not sure what to think, either. I guess time will tell. I feel confident that he didn't have a stroke yesterday, but going forward . . . that's why I have to recommend you take it easy. You're still on the blood thinners, and I'm going to prescribe something for your headaches that will help with depression too. There are the usual side-effects—constipation, nausea—but it should help more than it hurts."

"Okay. Thanks," was all I could muster.

"You're one for the books, Kevin. From a medical standpoint your story is incredible. Your arm, the blood clots—all this might have truly disabled you, but here you are."

"Here I am," I answered, to fill the silence. *Truly* disabled. He had no idea how brittle my brain felt and how strung out I was. Like most doc-tors, he knew the effects on paper, but there was no way I could show them inside my head to see the wrestling matches among my neurons, fighting for balance and stability, jockeying for position in a forest of felled synapses. When I looked at Sam the doctor disappeared into my blind spot. If only I could accomplish the same magic with my symptoms.

The doctor continued, "Someone should write a paper on this. It is very rare for someone of your age and physicality to have this happen to you, to have an aneurysm, much less endure strokes. I would guess something like one in seventy-five million."

Wow, I thought. *How lucky am I?*

But this was no time for sarcasm. I was too busy worrying about giving up the movie, losing the nice paycheck, and giving in to the tiny angry devils in my head that were destroying me. I hated this. I hated hospitals, doctors, nurses, blood, and feeling like I had no choice in my life anymore. My brain steadfastly refused to straighten out and behave normally. It was like a disobedient, spoiled child. Like Chuckie, with the red hair and scarred face.

I was at his mercy.

After two days the Crawford Long Hospital in Atlanta released me on my own recognizance. It was my birthday, September 24, but I was not celebrating.

I had spoken to a number of people from the *Black Dog* set. Meat Loaf had even called me in the hospital. They were shooting some scenes I wasn't in and some stunt stuff as well, scrambling to keep the crew working without the star of the show.

They were all encouraging me to "feel better."

I answered that I was "working on it."

It was "depressing."

One of the producers on the show, Ben, came to visit Sam and me in the apartment to give me a birthday gift. He, too, was supportive. "This is a minor setback in your life, Kevin. They've scrambled to keep shooting without you while you heal, so take your time now and enjoy your birthday. You'll be back in no time." Somehow, his every encouragement layered on more doubt.

Very early in my modeling career I worked with a guy named Chris, a photographer in Dallas who was openly gay. I'm straight. No big deal. I view sexuality as a private matter and I respect people's privacy.

I was doing a bathing-suit shoot with two gorgeous female models. "Beautiful, that's right. Cammi, lean back a little more. Perfect! Lisa, turn your chest more this way. Show those ta-tas! Great! Kevin, never mind! You're *perfect!* Ha ha! Okay, laughing and having fun, children!" He was snapping photos, the flashes going. "Okay, ladies—and boy! Ha ha! We got that one. Let's get changed into your next suits—and I don't mean your *birthday suits!*" He was a bit crass, but the job paid well.

I changed into a Speedo-type suit in navy and purple, and I was back on set, a tacky beach scene against a white backdrop. I was standing barefoot in the sand next to a beach chair and umbrella as Chris came over to hand me a beach ball.

"You're a really good model, Kevin. You have the perfect package—for modeling, you know? Great looks, plus you move really well for the camera . . ."

Wow, I thought. "Thanks," I said. Honestly, he was standing a little too close, and I was all but naked.

"How long have you been modeling?"

Okay, now, I could tell a come-on when I saw one. "For a few months. My girlfriend got me into it. You may know her . . ."

That's when I felt his hand on my ass, cupping it. I'm not normally a violent guy, but I do have very quick reactions, and before I knew what happened, I had slugged him and he went down.

When he came to, Chris was pretty upset. (He was gay, not masochistic.) He fired me on the spot and reported me to the agency. My booker, Gary, sat me down to discuss the incident. "Kevin, it's fine if you aren't gay, but you can't go hitting guys who come on to you," he told me.

"I know, Gary, but he grabbed my ass. It was a knee-jerk reaction. He violated my personal space." I knew Gary would appreciate the psycho-babble, but frankly, I was surprised at how easily it came to me. In any case, he responded well. "Yeah, I get that, violated. But punching the guy is still a little extreme, and you lost a client along with all of his future clients. You need to control your reactions. Can you do that?"

Gary was right. I agreed to keep my fists down if and when another situation like this came up.

It wouldn't be long. Once I got over to Europe, I became one of the new boys in town—"fresh meat," so to speak. I improved at fending off unwanted advances, gritting my teeth while choosing between *flattered* and *annoyed*. Often, a job was on the line, the modeling industry's version of the casting couch. Although *annoyed* usually won, I learned to candy coat it in a grace a Baryshnikov would be proud of. "I apologize for any misunderstanding," I'd say, and casually walk away, preserving dignity and ego for both of us.

I needed all that practiced patience to keep from lashing out against this new adversary and all the well-meaning but ignorant cheerleaders. I had a friend from set who suggested I scream into a pillow to exorcize my demons. I just nodded and thanked him for the advice.

"Things look bleakest before the dawn, Kevin. But the worst is over. Now you just have to rest and let nature take its course."

"Yes, of course. Thanks." The producer in Atlanta meant well, but his encouragement unwittingly provoked me into being more realistic about my illness.

"Hey, when you get down, what do you have to do?" Even just his energy exhausted me. He saw my blank look.

"Get back up again!" he finished, grinning. "You're Hercules, man! You can beat this thing! Plus, it's your birthday. This is no time to be sad, kiddo." I appreciated the sentiment, but inside, I twisted in a different knowledge; that infernal ache at the back of my head constantly reminded me, "This isn't over, yet—not by a long shot."

I padded around the apartment in bare feet and old sweats, too sick to walk but too anxious to sit. I wanted out of this disaster of a body. I desperately needed to just be the old me, the fast, determined, dedicated me—to turn back time, sit up on Dr. Hank's table, and say, "That's enough on the neck, now . . . no cracking!" My insides screamed. My body craved a workout, but my exhausted, confused, and very, very sad brain intervened with a resounding *NO*.

Sam held the door as Raffaella gingerly entered my apartment. "Oh, you are walking around. This is a good sign, yes?" Her quiet, lilting Italian accent could not soothe my aggravation.

I stood at the window overlooking the vast greenery below, taking in the separation and utter loneliness I felt, gazing out on the world I was no longer a part of. I wished I could blast my fist through that pane of glass and shatter my nightmare. I turned and perched on the sill.

"Well, I'm not dead yet, I guess."

I was trying to make a joke, but it didn't come out that way. Too soon?

Raffaella crossed the room to me to kiss both my cheeks. "Let's talk, okay?" She motioned to the couch and we all sat down.

"Kay-vin, you are not doing too good. I can see that. This is not my decision, but I believe you need to rest. It is very serious, what happened to you." She had a gentle, loving manner. I liked her so much. In that moment on the couch, she embodied honesty, belief in me, and quiet strength. "What do you think?"

Her obvious candor encouraged that same quality in me. "Raffaella, I'm so sorry. The last thing I want to do is pull out of this movie. I want to finish it. I need to work." My eyes got wet with frustration. I just wished I could *work*, work *out*, work *things* out.

I looked at Sam. She was uncharacteristically quiet, and she looked sorrowful. It hit me in that moment that this was a turning point. If I backed away from this fight, I would be branded a coward—certainly in my own mind, and maybe in Sam's too, but also, most probably, by an unforgiving, fickle industry. My movie career was now in jeopardy, big time. *Hercules* was cruising the world as a massive hit television show. It gave me *Kull*, my first lead in a feature. That gave me this movie, *Black Dog*. Backing out was going to derail my momentum, push me to the back of the line. I struggled fifteen years to get here, poised for action stardom, and now it would all disappear. I felt sick to my stomach. I was disgusted, too, from the realization that work was my main concern. Here I was, lucky to be alive, and all I could think about was my professional future.

"I don't want to let you down, Raffaella. I know what you went through to get this movie green lit for me. I know."

Raffaella shrugged off my compliment. "Kay-vin, the most important thing is your health. I think you need some time to heal. You remember how sick I was during filming of *Kull* last year? I do not want that for you. It is not good for you, especially as an actor. And it is not good for the movie. But if you think you can do the movie, then I trust you. So. What do you think, eh?"

I flushed. The droning sound in my head was back with a vengeance. Ever since I collapsed on set, all my symptoms seemed amplified, like pit bulls locked on their prey. I leaned forward into my nausea, putting my face in my clammy hands.

"Kay-vin," she stroked my back, "I can find another actor for the role. I do not want to, but it can be done. And insurance is already computing for the adjustment. There is nothing for you to worry about. You just need to tell me what you want to do, darling."

My fight floated away on her sincerity. Inside, I lowered my fists. I kept my head down and admitted softly, "I can't do the movie, Raffaella. I just can't."

She hugged my back, speaking softly. "I know, darling. I know. You are doing the right thing. I want you to go get some rest and stop trying to kill yourself. Your body, I know, is tired of all your hard work. Don't worry about this little crap movie. Get your health back and then worry about the movies."

Her advice was quite reasonable, but I railed against reason. I saw everything that I had worked for slipping away.

Quitting the movie meant failure. I threw my clothes into my suitcase, feeling like I was throwing my life in there with them—packing it up into storage.

I was hopeless and down. And I was confused too. *Could I really be this sick?* Clearly, there was an issue inside my head. *Three strokes, for real?* I wasn't even forty yet! In a single heartbeat, I had transformed from a youthful, carefree jock into a failing octogenarian—grasping onto countertops and chair backs for an arduous five-yard trip to the bathroom. How could this be?

But my pounding, throbbing, humming brain whispered to me, "It's my turn. I'm running the show now."

I couldn't even nod my head in capitulation. It hurt too much.

TOO MUCH WORK

Sam Sorbo

I WAS NEWLY IN LOVE when I boarded the flight back to Los Angeles, elated and anxiety ridden. I believed I had possibly met the man of my dreams, but I was not so wide-eyed and naive as to trust my senses. Did "love at first sight" truly exist? It would take some time for me to be assured of that.

I had spent my final days in Auckland searching for the problem, the caveat, the one issue that would spell doom for our relationship. What on earth was wrong with Kevin Sorbo? So far, nothing I could find.

I thought back to when he picked me up in his Ford Taurus the previous Saturday night for our first real date. "Wow!" I remarked, "You listen to country music?"

He reached for the dial. "Oh, we can change that if you want to . . ."

"No, no! I love country music. Don't change it." I smiled to myself. He was a gentleman and a cowboy.

Now, relaxing on the plane, I wondered about our future. He would be passing through LA in two weeks, and I would see him then. Oh! I wanted to see him right away! Two weeks is such a long time for a budding romance to sit idle.

Before meeting Kevin I had eagerly been pursuing my acting career, and what I dreamed of more than anything was having my own TV show. I felt like I had the talent, drive, and smarts to pull it off. (How little I knew back then!)

After watching Kevin at work for nearly two weeks, I recognized the extraordinary commitment that a TV drama—that Hercules—demanded. I sat in my Air New Zealand seat, reflecting on him working: memorizing the fight choreography, pacing off-set while learning his lines for upcoming scenes, studying scripts over lunch, pushing weights at the gym. Watching him prepare and rehearse was poetry. I witnessed how incredibly adept he was at it all, but his time was hardly his own; his life was nonstop.

"Well, I don't want my own show, that's for sure," I whispered to myself. "That's way too much work."

It turns out I was right.

It was too much work, even for Hercules.

MOURNING

IT'S BEEN THREE DAYS since I sacrificed the movie and boarded a plane back to LA from Atlanta. I've been laying low in Sam's condo, trying to re-organize, figure out what to do and where to go next, and make some sense of my life these days.

Tomorrow I have yet another MRI, this one to assure us that my episode in Atlanta had not caused more damage. I'm not looking for-ward to the clanging metal on my brain. Admitting I am sick is one thing, but every new appointment, every new medical procedure ce-ments in my mind the uncertainty of my situation. I have to get off the couch, but I have no energy. I am not sleeping well at night, and I often wake up sweating.

Stop being so f-ing lame, I decide. I almost go for the elevator, but I browbeat myself over to the stairwell instead. Gripping the banister and berating myself the entire way, I climb the stairs of Sam's refined 1980s building to the roof, six stories above the street. The steel door gives onto black asphalt and a mediocre terrace with green carpeting amid several untidy planters.

I am alone with my thoughts, my regrets, and my health issues. Pre-occupied as I am with my symptoms, the cool air soothes my frazzled nerves enough for me to calm my breath and glance around. The wake-ful city zips about below: cars moving into parking spaces, people laughing as they walk by on the sidewalk, and a late-night TV show drifts through an open window in the building next door. Life goes on.

A murky night sky hovers overhead, with stars twinkling through like so much Hollywood glitter. And there is the moon, my old friend. "Moon" was my first word, I'm told—and my first love. I used to gaze, entranced, at her luminous magnificence. She ruled the sky.

But tonight, through my tears, I see only a small white disk, a paper plate as distant from the earth as I am from myself. I feel as though I am in mourning. I have lost a close friend—the guy I used to be.

THE GOOD NEWS

SAM AND I ARE HEADED TO CHURCH, mainly because Sam requires it. I never had a chance to visit Sam's church when I was healthy—I guess I was never in town long enough—so this is our first opportunity to worship together, and I have to at least give her that.

Don't get me wrong: My good Christian parents raised me in the Lutheran church and I am a believer. But I am also kind of ticked off at the Big Guy. I need someone to blame for what happened to me, and God was in the wrong place at the right time. Going to His house was not really on my to-do list. Then again, I reason, I need all the help I can get.

Christian Assembly is an unassuming, squat stucco building that looks a little crushed under its wide low-pitched roof. What the small, mustard-and-brown amphitheater lacks in panache, however, the congregation more than makes up for in personality.

As we walk into the sanctuary the lilting strains from Tommy Walker's guitar and the rest of the five-piece band buoys me. Tommy is a renowned worship leader, combining a self-effacing humor with innate musical aptitude. He also has a fantastic voice, and when the choir joins in, it puts a soft smile in my heart. I tamp my emotions down as best as I can. There are eyes on me. *Hercules is at our church!* I can hear them through my skin.

I feel shaky. But then again, when don't I feel shaky these days?

The Friday before, back at Cedars for more tests, had been difficult, and my symptoms were retaliating. I think back to Dr. Bookman's relentless, *stupid* neurological testing: Flip the hand, stand on one foot, follow my finger with your eyes. Just because I could execute those silly hand gestures didn't prove I was anywhere near *my* normal. My (former athlete's) performance was severely compromised—something the doctor couldn't seem to appreciate. I wrestled with my faulty balance while he made notes and grunts.

I had asked him, point blank, why he sent me back to work on the movie, why he thought I could handle it, knowing what he did of my injuries. "Well, you're Hercules," he answered with a twinkle in his eye and a shrug of the shoulders.

Incredulous, I countered, "You know that's a TV show, right? I'm not really half-god. I'm an actor." I did not have a twinkle.

"Well, Kevin, your first MRI didn't show any strokes, so we couldn't know that for sure. We had very limited ways to confirm the extent of the damage. You seemed okay at the time—a little shaken, maybe. You look fine now, and you're walking and talking, so . . ."

I thought about my own complicity in denying my injuries. The studio didn't want my image tarnished, but neither did I. More than that, I flatly refused to recognize my fragility. That a few tiny clots might sideline me was offensive and unacceptable.

"But I told you I was dizzy, nauseated, that I felt shaky. And the lightning strikes behind my eyelids . . ."

"Well, you did have a brush with death, Kevin, and that's a traumatic event. Remember, we also discussed how much better you felt," he smiled. "Look, I can't get inside your head. I thought you were well enough to work."

"Why didn't you tell us the strokes wouldn't even *be* on the MRI, though?" Sam was just as frustrated as I was with this seeming catch-22, while he tried to be charming.

He shrugged. "Look, there is no reason to make more of something . . . technically, they're ministrokes . . ." He, too, wanted to make little of the assault on my brain. But he was wrong, as I had been.

"There is nothing *mini* about these things, doctor."

In the church my heart pounds along with the swelling music. Its energy courses through my body. There had been a time, recently, when I thrived on this kind of rush. Not any longer. My head starts throbbing.

The song ends, and Tommy opens with a short prayer and then starts gently strumming his guitar, the chords settling on the reverent crowd like a cozy morning fog.

> *I have a father*
> *He calls me his own*
> *He'll never leave me*
> *No matter where I go*
> *He knows my name*
> *He knows my every thought*
> *He sees each tear that falls*
> *And hears me when I call*

I lose my inner battle; my tears fall silently in my lap.

My Father had whispered to me, "Don't let him crack your neck." Twice I heard that warning and had failed to act upon it. Why warn me? Why let it happen? Why, God, why? My questions keep time with the music.

The song finishes and the pastor, Mark Pickerill, begins to speak. I like him immediately. I am accustomed to the preacher in the pulpit throwing down warnings like lightning bolts, cautioning about God's wrath. Mark is an entirely different kind of messenger, with more enticing ideas about God along with a healthy sense of humor. I listen with interest as he describes a loving Savior who seeks our hearts. Although my soul is heavy, for the first time, I feel validated in church.

After church Sam and I exit the sanctuary. The throng of joyful people greeting each other inadvertently stalls our exit, and a boy in a wheelchair approaches me. "Mr. Sorbo? Hercules? Could I get a picture with you, please?"

How can I refuse a sweet child in a wheelchair? His dad shoots a happy photo of us, with me on one knee, leaning over to put my face near his. The flash catches people's attention. Most people had probably thought not to trouble me for an autograph in church, but this gives them license.

They all see me as Hercules, not sick or weak or vulnerable. I refuse to disappoint them. The relationship an actor has with an iconic character like mine is intense. (I'm not saying it's healthy.) When Charles Barkley says in the Nike commercial, "I am not a role model," he denies the mantle of responsibility that accompanies everyone who reaches that certain level of notoriety. Though it is true that he does not get paid to be a role model, one cannot refuse the honor just by speaking out against it. It is sewn into the fabric of fame.

By the time we make our way outside the church, Sam and I are surrounded, and I manage a forty-five-minute autograph session.

"I read about your aneurysm. I know they fixed it, so you're okay now?"

"You look thinner, Kevin. But you're feeling better now, right?"

"I saw the reports on *ET!* Thank God you came through it. You're awesome, and we watch your show religiously! Oops! Can I say that in church?" Ha ha ha.

That my fans choose *Hercules*—and me by default—is an incredible tribute, but an unavoidable by-product of television is that they see us as a single unit. I do not have the courage or arrogance enough to reject their admiration—certainly not today. But my mantle has recently become quite heavy. I am not really the hero they think I am anymore. I feel entirely conflicted.

Adding injury to insult, my brain begins to retaliate. Sam and I extricate ourselves from the group; I grab her arm to help me not fall over. I need to sit down, and I am petrified of having an episode in front of all these witnesses. Keeping my more serious health issues a secret was difficult, especially in light of a second hospitalization. When we finally get to her car, I push my seat all the way back, recline it, and shut my eyes. Luckily, Sam knows me well enough not to talk: I have one of my "migraines" setting in.

Although sometimes strokes pass and take their temporary damage with them, like with my impaired speech, my eyesight had not noticeably improved over those first few weeks of recovery. "The brain frequently learns to adjust," the doctors told me. *Terrific.* When I looked far left or right, my eyeballs twitched, and I had constant "lightning flashes," intense displays of electric-like pulses behind my closed eyes. Reading was out of the question. When I started at the top of the page, the right part would be blank. As I read across, more lines would appear, as if by magic. Now you see them, now you don't.

I had no respite from the dizziness, nausea, and the searing pains and aches in my head, arm, and chest. I constantly felt like I was falling backward, and I often jolted to catch myself even though I wasn't moving. It was an unnerving though logical consequence of my particular brain damage.

Tinnitus, an often inexplicable ringing in the ears, has been known to drive people crazy. That unrelenting generator sound at the base of my skull was my own version of this phenomenon: constant and maddening, drowning out any coherent thoughts and destroying my sleep. I wanted to believe it was my brain trying to sort itself out, but my doctors wouldn't confirm that hypothesis. Another weird symptom: I would smell an almond odor, for no apparent reason. "Phantom smells are a fairly common side effect of strokes," one of the doctors explained.

The strokes had clearly brought these symptoms on, but the docs didn't know when (or if) they would cease. In these early days their lack of answers was terribly aggravating. I sought another opinion.

Dr. Weissman, the head of neurology at a prestigious nearby medical center, was a pillar of the medical community and came highly recommended. This was just after the enormous fiasco in Atlanta, my collapsing on set; Sam and I entered his small office with high hopes. The doctor sat behind his pale wooden desk, backed by a bursting bookcase, and we gamely took the two chairs facing him.

Weissman was a kind gentleman with a soft, reassuring manner. After his exam he gave us an overview of my type of issues, speaking easily in frank tones. "Kevin, the good news is that physically, your body is very healthy. Your movements are good and reflexes strong. But you have injured your brain, and that is serious business. The nystagmus, the involuntary rapid eye movement, is not terribly pronounced, and it should go away. This and the vision loss are probably contributing to your headaches, so you can reasonably expect those to improve over time. You have some residual weakness and control issues in your left arm, and these, too, should resolve favorably. The dizziness and nausea might also dissipate, but only time will tell. After three months most of the improvement should be complete."

Three months. Good news. I was feeling like I was dying, so three months sounded like a really awesome deal.

"Exactly how much improvement you can expect is indeterminate," he continued. "For instance, typically, vision loss does not heal, but the brain learns to adjust. But you must allow it time. You've been living a very unhealthy lifestyle, with the lack of adequate sleep, and driving yourself too hard. I must point this out, Kevin: You have suffered a serious, life-altering illness. You should not take that lightly."

Yeah, yeah, yeah. *Three months* was ringing in my ears; I didn't hear any of that other stuff.

"Kevin, I'm going to recommend no work for five weeks. You're on hiatus now, is that right?"

"Yes, until early November."

He consulted his notes. "Right, I see. I think we need to tell them to give you another week off. And when you do go back to work, only a limited work schedule. Ease back into it. I'm going to prescribe a higher dose of the blood thinners and a vasodilatory agent to combat the headaches, which seem to be vascular in nature. You aren't a clotter, right?"

Ugh. My head was spinning, from the buzzing as much as the thought of not working out for weeks. "Right," Sam answered for me.

He confirmed it on his notes. "Yes, here it is. So those prescriptions will both be temporary. Eventually, though, if your vertigo does not improve on its own, we'll get you into physical therapy.

"One final point: I'd like to get another study done on your neck to determine the cause of the strokes. It is implausible that they were related to the aneurysm, frankly, and I'd like to confirm that they came from the neck twist. Most commonly it would be a C1-C2 rotational issue, although the placement of the lesions is not compatible with this mechanism, but it might also be an intervertebral spur. If it isn't either of those, then it must be an embolic phenomenon, in which case we need to be treating that in order to prevent reoccurrence. I'm also recommending another agent that will screen against this being a syndrome instead of a singular event tied in with the chiropractic adjustment. I don't think you are in danger anymore, but I need the study results to be certain."

"Okay," I answered, a little off-balance from the barrage of information. I wasn't sure how to process that he also didn't believe the aneurysm with the neck-twist caused the strokes. Could I still have some other rogue culprit inside me, waiting to lob more clots at my brain? I certainly felt like I was yet under siege.

"Finally, Kevin, you need to understand you have had a systemic illness, and your fatigue—the sleeping long hours—is completely normal for this type of thing. Your sleep patterns were highly unusual *before* this happened. Your body needs rest."

"Right," I capitulated.

"That's the good news, though. You *can* rest." He smiled.

"Yes, I can," I repeated back, a meaningless mantra. "What about exercise?"

He shook his head. "No gym, no weight lifting. You can go for walks or ride a stationary bike, but you need rest more than anything. I'm going to advise you only an hour walk each day. From there, you can build back up, but no lifting for at least a month or more." His look was stern and compassionate at the same time. "Did you have any other questions for me?"

"Just one," I said. "Sam and I were also wondering about our wedding, if you thought we should postpone it or what we should do." I looked at her.

"I'm leery of adding more stress on top of this," she explained.

His answer was immediate and direct. "I tell people never to put life on hold for an illness."

I will never forgive him for that!

Just kidding . . .

With Dr. Weissman's blessing, for both the wedding and the timing of my recuperation, we decided to start planning.

BUILDING A BRIDGE

I WAS IN MY EARLY TWENTIES and in Italy for only a short while when my Milanese modeling agents, Beatrice Models [pronounced *Bay-ah-trree-chay*] sent me on a go-see to Gianni Versace's. They were sure he would love me.

A go-see is a two- or three-hour time slot when invited models show their books, making small talk while the photographer or art director pages through their portfolios. They are usually cattle calls, with lots of bored-looking models hanging around, waiting their turns. Modeling is such an odd business. "Hi. Here are pictures of me. Aren't I great? Please book me. Please."

In the '80s, the average male model was a lot smaller than me. Five–foot-ten to six feet tall was the norm, 38–40 regular. I came in at almost six-foot-four and a 46 long jacket, but my agent told me my height would be a bonus for fashion shows because the women in heels were all over six feet tall.

On the appointed day the place was filled with male models all hoping for the great Versace to pick them for his fashion show. Into the mad throng of the waiting room, a door flew open and Gianni saw me from inside his office. Italians wave you in a little differently. Instead of the large American gesture of raising an upturned palm and pulling it toward you, Italians put out a downturned palm and then simply drop the fingers to indicate, "Come!" This is how Gianni called to me, ignoring both protocol and his protesting assistant, Marco (who had already turned me down twice before).

I sat opposite Gianni in his sumptuous office. He took a moment to peruse my book. "Kay-vin Sorrrrbo," he said, smiling through his heavy accent. "Why have I not seen you before?" I shrugged and suggested he ask Marco. Gianni frowned. "I like your look. Iz good for my show. I will see you again there, Kay-vin," he said, smiling.

In the show with me was a Brazilian guy named Max. He was tall, like me, and really good looking. But unlike many models I knew, he was totally cool—a real person who was easy to relate to. He regarded modeling as a great business opportunity, not a life calling.

Max pulled me aside during the show and said, "Kevin, you have something fantastic here. Fantastic. You must keep your eyes open and you will see. This will be fantastic for you."

I didn't get it. I looked at him quizzically, and he continued, "Gianni really likes you. He needs someone for his next campaign. You play it right, that could be you."

Now, campaigns are the Holy Grail for models because they are exclusivity contracts—guaranteed work, great exposure, and, of course, a nice payday. We all wanted campaigns.

After the show I went out with a couple friends for dinner and a beer, called it a night, and went home. I was reading a book in bed when my phone rang.

"*Pronto.*"

"*Ciao*, Kay-vin, iz Gianni."

"Gianni, who?"

"Kay-vin! Iz Gianni Versace."

"Oh! Hi, Gianni. Um, what can I do for you?"

"I want to invite you to a party tonight. I send a car. You come."

"Oh, I'm sorry, but I'm really tired . . ."

"No, no. You come. The car is already coming to pick you up. Iz good."

He got my home number from my agent, of course. Let me explain: The agent works for both the model and the client, taking commissions from both. (Conflicts of interest be damned.) Now, who has more career longevity? The client does, so in general, the client gets the loyalty.

Therefore, if the client asks for a phone number . . . Usually it would be to set up young female models with Italian playboys. (Oh, if those parents only knew this when they send their fourteen- to nineteen-year-olds over to model in Italy, with the agents' promise that their daughters would be "well taken care of.")

Back to Gianni. My curiosity overcame my fatigue, so I went to the party. In short order I was introduced to Sophia Loren, Pavarotti, Madonna, and Richard Gere. The list went on and on. I was in a dream world. Versace's place was a breathtaking, grand-scale, old Milano building built for a different century, with high ceilings and columns in the living room. The carpets and furnishings were all in the Versace style, of course, so everywhere I turned there were spectacular things to look at—I mean, in addition to the guests. Contributing to the entertainment, Elton John played piano for a bit. The whole thing was surreal.

The next evening Gianni called again to say that a car would be coming to bring me to another party. Of course, I went. Why not? This time, the car dropped me off for a smaller dinner party of twelve guests. Great food and wine, and to say it was very nice would be an understatement. I chatted, enjoying the openness of the Italian culture and the expressiveness, passion, and humor in their boisterous conversations. (The way Italians use their hands for emphasis when they speak has always fascinated me.) The company was friendly and entertaining, and Gianni made a wonderful host. At the end of the evening I thanked him for the invite and went home.

Not long after that Versace called again. I reminded myself that this was a business opportunity, so I joined him at an intimate, refined restaurant, and it turned out that although we were seated at a table for four, it would be just the two of us dining. We were sitting catty-corner to each other, having a lively discussion about life, when Gianni's hand came to rest on my thigh. I gently removed it and smiled at my uneasy predicament.

I said, affably, "Gianni, come on. You know I am straight."

Gianni quickly picked up the thread with his characteristic charm and candor. "Of course! This is why I like you. You are not a girly man. You are a man!"

I laughed. "Gianni, you know that 'this' will never happen. Sorry, but I'm a *flaming* heterosexual."

Gianni chuckled amiably but continued, "Kay-vin, in life you must try everything. In sex, too, you must try—with a woman, with a man, with a dog and a goat. You must try everything and experience the entire world."

I looked at him for a moment before I reasoned, "Gianni, all my life, I've been on this road." I gestured a flat pavement with my palm down. "And you, you're traveling on this road," gesturing with my other hand out, palm down. I looked at him, shrugging at the impossibility of the situation.

As quick as a wink, he reached across both of my hands and said, "I build a bridge!"

I have to say, I laughed out loud, and I have never forgotten it. Although I never did get the Versace campaign, we remained friends, and I continued to do his shows. It was a sad day when I heard the news of his death. He was a very bright, talented, charming man.

After resigning the movie in Atlanta and landing back in LA with my tail between my legs, it was finally sinking in that this illness had kicked my ass, forced me to quit a big picture deal, and lay me down like a featherweight on the floorboards screaming, "Uncle!" I needed a way back from that impossible humiliation, and I needed some more answers to quell my anger and frustration.

I needed to build a bridge, and I knew just the place to start construction.

In 1994 the studio decided to make a TV series out of *Hercules*. After the first five movies I looked at my 1993 tax return and saw that I was paying the state of California 10 percent of my earnings even though I was really living seven thousand miles away in New Zealand.

I called Beverlee and asked her to find me a place in Las Vegas, Nevada. I loved the desert mountains reaching up to the cloudless blue sky—that and the absence of a state income tax. Bev sent me pictures of some options, and I picked a place in Henderson, Nevada, on a golf course. (Surprised?)

It was south of the strip, in the newest, fastest growing part of the blossoming city. I closed on the three-bedroom townhouse from the distant confines of my pad in Auckland. It turned out to be one of the few smart investments I have ever made.

When I bought the place there was only one—unfinished—road out that way, and my development sat at the end of it. The condo was a cookie-cutter with a decent floor plan. The carpeting was aqua, and the furnishing, done on the fly during a quick trip back home, was pine and beige, straight off the showroom floor. The view out the living room window was of a small grassy area overlooking the golf fairway. Green, green, and more green. My new home wasn't anything too special, not a big place by any means, but it was comfortable, functional, and mine.

And it was quiet—just what I needed now. Sam and I unpacked and settled in for the recovery period.

~~~

Three months. Ninety days. Twelve weeks until I was done "improving." They told me not to overexert myself, to take it easy. What did that mean? I had never taken it easy in my life. I had five more weeks of hiatus, including the extra week off, but I had no idea how to begin to heal.

During those first days back home I sat on the couch, running through my list of afflictions while Sam prepared dinner. I wasn't trying to be morbid; I was just sizing up my opponent. Television was my only distraction, but there is only so much television a person can take, frankly, so I often simply lay on the couch contemplating my navel. Again and again, I wondered *why*: Why must I feel like a Mack truck had run me down twice? Why had God done this to me? Was I being punished? What for? Was there any hope? Was it going to be like this for the rest of my life? What if it gets worse?

Stroke and brain trauma are intimately linked, with two of the most common side effects being depression and mood swings, or anger. To combat these issues my doctors prescribed Buspar, Zoloft, Lexamil, Prozac, and more over the course of time. Although I felt like a pharmacy, like a good little boy I tried—and eventually eliminated—each one.

I had been on Buspar, for instance, for over two weeks, and I hated the way I was feeling. Buspar slowed everything down. I was in a hurry, impatient. I needed some fast relief, some immediate healing. I concluded that Buspar was hindering my recovery—or at least my attitude: It was preventing me from being me.

I called the doctor and explained that I felt worse on the drug than off it, and he argued that often it takes a while for the drug to work. I relented for another week, but then my patience was taxed, and I went off of it. Believe it or not, I actually felt even worse. I called him back and told him, and he suggested I try the drug again. *Yeah, right.* I asked if it might be withdrawal. The doctor did not believe so, but Sam quickly called the pharmacist, who confirmed it probably was.

The side effects of most mood-altering drugs are listed as constipation, decreased appetite, decreased sex drive, diarrhea, dizziness, dry mouth, headache, nervousness, and drowsiness. Then there are the less frequent offerings, such as seizures, hallucinations, shortness of breath, muscle cramps, and suicidal thoughts. Of course, given my new outlook, my expectations for their efficacy were extremely low. That seemed to pan out. None of the drugs I tried offered me relief, only side effects— more of what I already had. They were prescribed to fend off the expected depression, but they only ended up making me more depressed.

I know it sounds contradictory, but I was still hoping for an instantaneous recovery, a miracle cure, and even though I didn't believe they would work, with each drug's failure, I sank deeper.

A LONG WALK SPOILED

About a month into my Nevada exile, Steve Wynn, the legendary Las Vegas developer, called to invite me to a celebrity golf tournament for CaP CURE, a charity dedicated to finding a cure for prostate cancer. I made some lame excuse about my shoulder still healing, but Steve wouldn't take no for an answer. He convinced me instead that an outing might be good for me.

Shadow Creek is a marvel of human imagination and engineering, a gorgeous Colorado golf course in the middle of the Nevada desert, with wandering peacocks and pheasants to complete its idyllic picture. Sam and I arrived about halfway through the tournament, and as we pulled up, Peter Jacobsen, the PGA tour player and a longtime friend, was making the turn. He greeted us warmly and asked how I was doing. I gave him the same line I had been practicing, rubbed my shoulder a bit to sell it, and then said, "But this is the most gorgeous course, so I couldn't just take a pass."

He laughed and said, "I know what you mean. It beckons you, right?"

"You have no idea!" Not being able to golf was enormously frustrating, but with my balance issues and poor sight, I couldn't even address the ball.

Sam and I got a cart and set out around the course. The tournament was a who's who of Hollywood golfing celebrities and a lot of fun. On the eleventh hole we discovered Greg Norman golfing with Kerry Packer, the billionaire Australian media mogul.

Packer had landed on a flat area, facing a steep upslope with a tree at the top. It was a very tough blind shot—no flag in sight. Against Norman's suggestion, Kerry determined to punch through the tree.

"Yes, sure, give it a try! Trees are 99 percent air, anyway." Norman brawled, winking at us.

Packer skulled his ball so hard that it stuck right into the hill, about twenty yards away.

There was a moment of surprise. Then Norman said, "Of course, *hills* are 100 percent solid . . ." We all laughed.

Norman threw down a ball and lobbed a shot directly over the tree at the top of the hill, smiled at Sam, and said, "That's what I was talking about." Norman's ball had landed two feet from the pin.

After golf there was a reception with an elaborate spread in the club lounge. Upholstered chairs, luxurious carpeting, and soft music created a muted ambiance conducive to conversation and relaxation. Sam and I mingled happily.

James Garner was seated at a table with Clint Eastwood, who called us over to tell me his little girl loved my series and would pronounce it "Percules." I was always amazed to find out who watched my show within the celebrity crowd!

Then I turned to Garner, reminding him that it was the second time that we were meeting. "I don't expect you to remember this, but I caddied for you twenty years ago at the Duff's Celebrity tournament in Minnesota."

He frowned first but then brightened. "Yes, of course! I remember Duff's." Then, with a glint in his eye, he asked, "Did I stiff you on the tip?"

I laughed. "Come to think of it, you did, and I'm here to collect!"

"You know, I think I do remember you, and your sarcastic sense of humor!" he answered, putting his arm around me. "I heard you were sick. You feeling better now?"

I lied, of course.

Actually, I was starting to feel a whole lot worse. Since leaving the course, all my symptoms had begun attacking with a vengeance, and they were reaching a crescendo. We left quickly, and by the time I got home I was feeling more ill than I ever had in the ICU.

I was confused and frustrated and depressed. My time had gone so well outside on the course. What had I done to be punished like this? I spent my next three days on the couch, panicked and losing hope, getting up only to go to the bathroom or to bed, and holding on to furniture to steady myself.

Over that time, as nothing worse came, the vice grip of my anxiety gradually loosened, and my symptoms eventually eased back to their baseline levels. Sam suspected that the (relative) confusion and cacophony at the event had been too much for my shattered brain to manage. Absurd, of course, but the doctors had no suggestions at all. For the first time since I got sick I realized that my reasoning and my will was no match for this thing, that even if I played by the rules, the rules might change, and then we'd be scrambling to figure it all out again.

But I was too bullheaded to actually give up the fight yet.

The walks in the mornings became my serene salvation. Autumn in Las Vegas is mild, with crisp dawns that submit leisurely to the arid desert sunshine.

Sam and I would have an unhurried breakfast and then head out for our hike. We chose an easy path. The city had required developers to build a kind of narrow side park along a canal behind their developments. From our townhouse we had to cross only a few streets to enter the green belt for a few miles.

Initially, our walks took barely an hour. I walked slowly. My balance was still not good, and the blind spot in my vision became more pronounced when I crossed blacktop streets. The flat, light-absorbing asphalt confused my brain, making it go crazy trying to focus and causing it to fall into a bottomless pit instead. The sensation was very odd, like a striped shirt that goes haywire on TV or when the horizontal goes wild and the entire screen flickers. To avoid it, at street corners I had to look to the sky. I felt like a weirdo.

Gizmoe came with us and enjoyed making the dogs behind the fences bark as we passed. Eventually, we increased the length and speed of our walks, and Gizmoe, who had an excellent memory for houses with dogs, would run ahead to get each dog riled up.

We started venturing farther. We crossed out of the residential area and into a business stretch, where we passed by a preschool every day. One day the kids saw us and came over to the fence. I saw a little boy with a crew cut—the very same cut I had had at his age. I elbowed Sam gently and said, "Hey, doesn't that little kid remind you of someone?"

"Yes," she answered. "You!"

It was true—he was a spitting image. I had found my mini-me. I called out to him as we passed and he answered with a wave.

"What's your name?" Sam asked.

The boy was not shy at all, holding to the tall fence with both hands. "Kevin!" he answered happily. "And this is my friend David!"

That was a bit freaky. Not only is my name Kevin, but David is my middle name. I stood below, on the concrete path, staring up at two cherubic little boys leaning with their hands casually hooked into the chain link fence. I tried picturing myself once being as they were just then: carefree and happy.

I used to be that young, that naive. I used to think the world was a great place, with incredible opportunity and wonderful adventures and places to explore, just for the asking. I used to live there.

My thoughts drifted in the hot, dry breeze, and they were unkind to me. *Look at the big picture that used to include you. It's not yours any longer.*

You are nobody and nothing.

Sam and I walked on in silence. It was a very long walk. Gizmoe was happy to get back home, and the rest of the day, as with every other day, she and I lazed on the couch, watching TV, listening to low music, or just having quiet time. I was blessed, actually, because the Brussels Griffon is like a toddler. They don't care what you are doing as long as they may join you.

Gizmoe was an effortlessly funny dog. With some pug in the breed, the Brussels Griffon has a pushed-in, monkey face and an inquisitive, loving nature. Because of her lack of a snout, Giz sneezed a great deal. Her snorts were often uncannily timed, seeming to indicate emphasis. She was headstrong and opinionated but affectionate to a fault. She might climb on you in her excitement to see you and then be so over-come that she snorts at you, expelling a fine mist of affection, which most people would call snot.

When Sam first told me about her small dog and showed me the photo, my initial reaction was, "That's not a dog, that's a rat!"

Sam, mildly offended, answered, "She's not a rat! She's actually a big dog in a small body." I was a hard sell. I never liked the yappy, snarling, trembling, purse-pets that small dogs always seemed to be. One day early in our relationship, I was visiting at Sam's condo in Beverly Hills, and I offered to take Giz for a quick walk. (I imagined this was a way to win points, both with Sam and the silly little rat-dog.) Sam gratefully handed me the leash, saying, "She'll just go far enough to do her busi-ness—end of the block, probably."

She had no idea. At first Giz simply refused to approach the door without Sam. She saw the leash and was excited to go outside—but not without Sam. My solution was to pick her up, carry her down the stairs, and bring her out the side door. I plunked her on some grass and she im-mediately squatted. I smiled. *Silly little dog, I knew you needed to go out-side for a walk!*

Once she finished I began to stroll and felt a tug on the other end of the leash. I looked back at her. She stood there on the sidewalk, defiant. I laughed out loud. "Yes, Giz, you weigh eight pounds, and you are going to stop me from pulling you down the street."

I tugged gently on the leash until she was forced to move. She walked four steps and dug in again, sitting in order to gain traction, her head pulled back, her front legs driven into the ground. She was rebellious, disallowing me from removing her from her rightful and distinguished role as protector of Sam. I pulled some more, hauling her from her stand, and she consented to walk a few more paces. Then she suddenly had had enough and started yanking on the leash, throwing her head back from side to side, pulling me back toward the door! I realized then that it would take more than a little pat on the head to win this dog's approval.

Lying on the couch for most of the day after a good, long, morning walk apparently made me alright in her eyes. She was always Sam's dog, but I like to think I earned a special place in her heart, because she certainly had one in mine. Her eight pounds of cuddly love and consolation offered me great comfort in my shaky condition. She would walk into the living room of my desert home and look around, snort or sneeze, and make me laugh. Then she would look at me as if to say, "What? What did I do that was so funny?" And I had to laugh again.

This little creature provided enduring support and comic relief. She's gone now, but as I write this, her memory yet floods me with warm affection for the big dog in the small body.

REHAB

THE DOCTORS PRESCRIBED REST, but I could not bear to sit idle and wait for some elusive peace treaty. Aside from my daily morning walks, I needed some action, a counterattack I could launch so I didn't feel so passive.

On doctor's advice, we signed me up for stroke therapy at a rehab center in Henderson. Sam drove me there. (I certainly couldn't.) The clinic was a spotless facility with treatment tables and work-out equipment that looked medieval in spite of their gleaming chrome.

Saul, my therapist, was a nice, well-built guy in his forties. He seemed competent and had a gentle, straightforward manner. He checked me in and took my history. Every time I told someone my story, it was hard. (Doing so is uncomfortable, to this day, but I have discovered it is also therapeutic.) People's incredulous reactions always made me feel more helpless. Even the professionals, who hid their initial surprise and approached treatment with positive words and a great attitude, could not disguise their uncertainty at treating a young person for an old guy's disease.

Ten percent of stroke victims recover almost completely; 15 percent die shortly after a stroke. Of all stroke sufferers, 40 percent need special care. Most importantly, though, only 28 percent are under age sixty-five. I was thirty-eight with three strokes—a complete anomaly. They could hazard guesses for my prognosis, but those were just that—guesses—and we both knew it.

Saul evaluated me with the typical undignified tests, like standing on one foot with my arms outstretched and touching my nose, and touching each of my fingers successively to the thumb of the same hand quickly and repeatedly. He asked me to walk on my toes and then my heels. I wasn't drunk, but my brain may as well have been. Many of these rudimentary tests I passed smoothly, if not effortlessly. Others, like bending over to touch my toes, were nearly impossible. I fell over the first time I tried it, and Saul gallantly caught me. Boy, that wasn't embarrassing at all.

Saul stood, appraising me. "I don't know what to do with you." He smiled like it was a compliment, but it didn't feel like one. "Let's start you with ball tosses. I want you to balance on this foot, catch with one hand, and keep one eye closed. Then we'll switch hands and do the same for the other foot."

I tried to smile. "Sure. Sounds like fun." It was more like mundane and stupid—and incredibly difficult. My progress was sluggish and I felt like a clown . . . a bad clown.

Eventually, I earned my way onto the balance boards. After that, Saul set me up in this box thing that was like a telephone booth with a wobbly floor. I tried to keep a red laser dot centered on a target by keeping my weight evenly balanced between my feet. My every move knocked it around. Breathing caused it to shift. To see how challenging standing still had become was extremely disconcerting, underlining my infirmity. How could I hit my mark and stay in focus if I couldn't do this simple thing?

At the end of the hour Sam would pick me up, sweaty and exhausted, with my brain feeling like mush. I'd return home to lie on the couch for the rest of the day with my nausea, vertigo, and a full-throttle buzzing at the back of my aching head. I could barely watch TV. Why was I not back on my feet yet? How was it possible I needed these people's help? I berated myself and wallowed in my degradation. Yeah, I was a ton of fun.

I had to go to rehab because it was the only thing I could do, but I was also terrified that it might do something to exacerbate my health issues.

The physicians didn't really know definitively why I experienced the strokes or if they might reappear. Each time I stood up, the dizziness and light-headedness hit me, and I would think, *This might be the time I just fall down for good.*

I was bluffing my way through each rehab session. Any day now my adversary could pick up his cards and go home, leaving me alone at the table with nothing. My only option was to gamble with everything I had, just to keep him interested. I was desperate to see this game to its natural finish, and I was equally determined to win. But I recognized I was playing against the house.

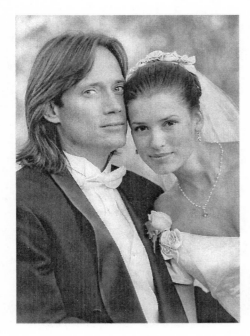

My wedding to Sam Jenkins, four months after my strokes, January 1998. *Photo by Joe Buissink*

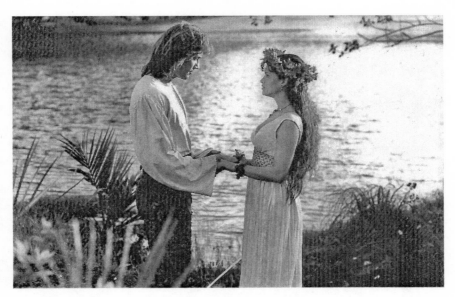

Art imitating life: Hercules marries Serena, December 1996. *Photo shot with my camera; Kevin Sorbo personal collection*

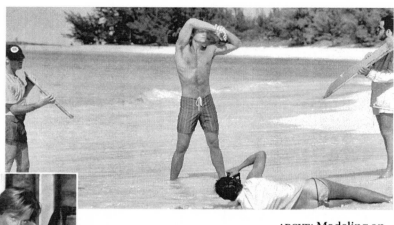

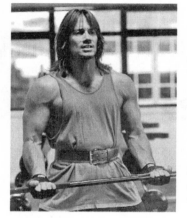

ABOVE: Modeling on the beach in the Bahamas, 1983. *Photo shot with my camera; Kevin Sorbo personal collection*

LEFT: Pumping iron in Auckland just months before the strokes, June 1997. *Photo by Pierre Vinet; Kevin Sorbo personal collection*

Shortly after arriving in Los Angeles, June 1986. *Photo by Kal Yee*

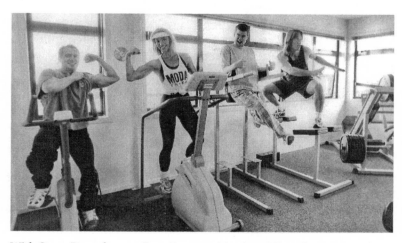

With Steve Rosenbaum, Cory Everson (six-time Miss Olympia), and Eric Gruendemann. *Photo by Pierre Vinet; Kevin Sorbo personal collection*

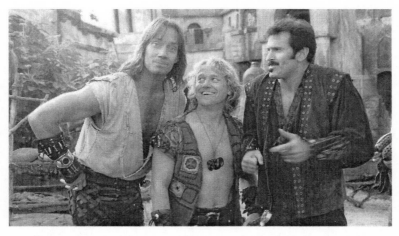

Goofing on the set with Michael Hurst as Iolaus and Bruce Campbell as Autolycus. *Photo shot with my camera; Kevin Sorbo personal collection*

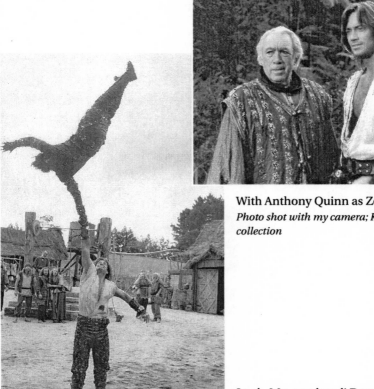

With Anthony Quinn as Zeus, 1994.
Photo shot with my camera; Kevin Sorbo personal collection

Look, Ma, one hand! December 1996.
Photo shot with my camera; Kevin Sorbo personal collection

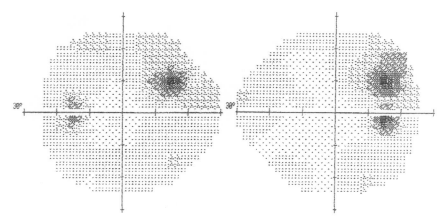

This is a map of my vision after the strokes. The dark spots represent vision loss, September 1997.

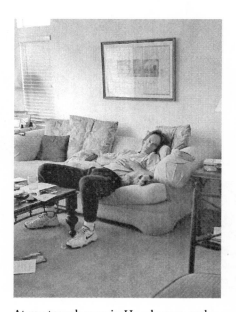

At my townhouse in Henderson, only weeks after the strokes. I wasn't doing too good, October 1997. *Photo by Sam Sorbo*

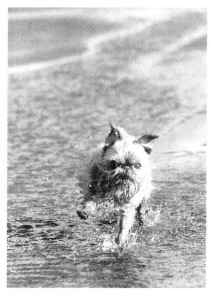

Giz loved running on sand. *Photo by Sam Sorbo*

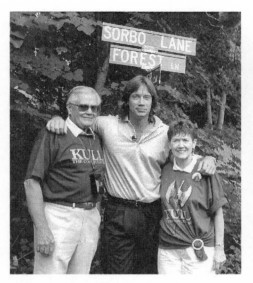

With Mom and Dad by the new Sorbo Lane sign, August 1997. *Photo by Diana Watters*

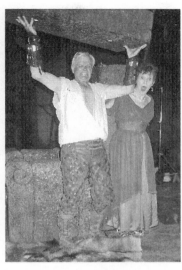

Mom and Dad muscling in on my turf, March 1996. *Photo by Kevin Sorbo*

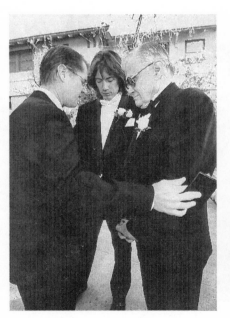

Dad, Pastor Mark, and me praying before my wedding. *Photo by Joe Buissink*

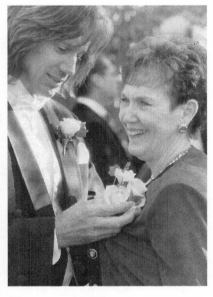

Mom at my wedding. *Photo by Joe Buissink*

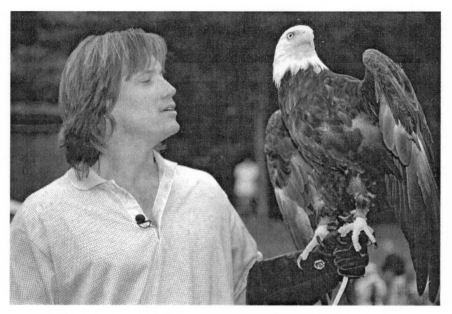

Posing with the University of Minnesota Raptor Center's tame eagle after releasing the rehabilitated one, 1997. *Photo by Diana Watters*

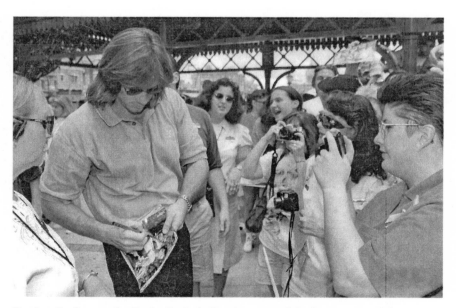

Signing for fans at the Sorbo Park dedication, a week before getting sick, August 1997. *Photo by Diana Watters*

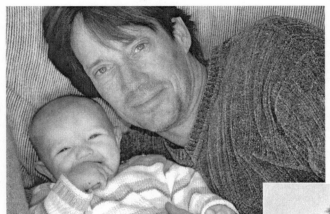

Me with Shane Haaken, my 12 ½-pound beast, Vancouver, 2004. *Photo by Sam Sorbo*

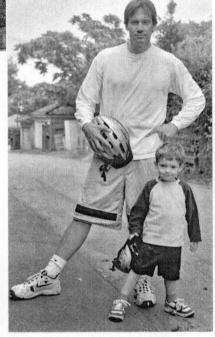

Dad and Braeden gear up for a bike ride, Vancouver, 2003. *Photo by Sam Sorbo*

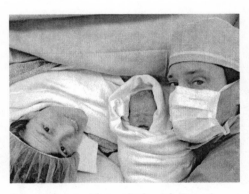

Sam and me with our little girl, Octavia Flynn. The prophecy fulfilled, Henderson, Nevada, 2005. *Photo by Kevin Sorbo*

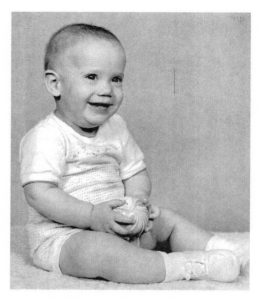

Wee baby Kevin. *Photo by Brenner Studio*

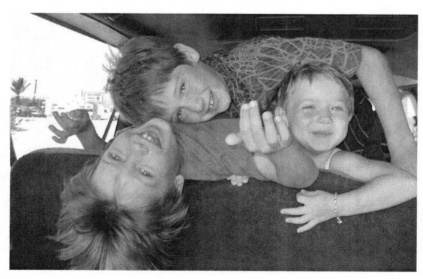

Three little miracles. *Photo by Sam Sorbo*

NO PARKING

The hottest club in town: Confetti's, Dallas, 1983.

I am the guy at the door. I work weekends only, twelve-hour shifts. I take the money for the cover charge, check IDs, flirt with the girls begging to get in, and greet all the Dallas Cowboy superstars when they descend for some fun: Tony Dorsett, Hollywood Henderson, Too-Tall Ed Jones, and Eric Dickerson, to name a few.

Inside, the place rocks. Loud, fast-paced dance music and pulsing lights filter through the hovering cigarette smoke. There are five bars split between two levels, several dance floors, and in cages built around fire poles and suspended between the levels, paid sexy dancers strut their stuff to the rhythm. Organized chaos.

One night the manager calls me outside at the door. "Kevin, there's a girl, topless, on the bar. Drunk, of course. Go get her down and get her out of here."

"Sure." I head inside, thinking, *Crap. Why'd he have to pick me?* But I already know: because I have the reputation of being able to talk people down from nasty situations.

A few months earlier Hollywood Henderson, the star linebacker for the Cowboys, came into the club for a fun evening. It was Halloween. The club went all-out and everyone was in costume. There was a bodybuilder, almost as wide as he was tall. He was dressed up as Bam-Bam,

Barney and Betty Rubble's baby in *The Flintstones*. He stood about five-foot-eight, but he was enormously built.

Hollywood measured more, though. At six-foot-three and 245 pounds, he was no slouch, either. But Bam-Bam was looking for a fight. He wanted to try to flatten one of the Dallas Cowboys' toughest players. Guys and their egos.

Bam-Bam was pestering Hollywood, saying he was "just a pussy," and "You think you're such a tough guy . . . come on, man, show me something, asshole. I could take you, you big faggot."

Hollywood was an easygoing guy and he wasn't looking for a fight, saying, "Look man, I don't know what your problem is. I'm just out with my friends . . ." But Bam-Bam wouldn't leave him alone, so Hollywood started engaging. The problem was that this punk was actually a threat. I mean this would be a big fight if someone didn't talk him down. I was minding my own business, taking cover charges inside, but it was all playing out a mere ten feet away from me, and it was starting to look ugly.

Into the fray I plunged. "Hi. I'm Kevin. What seems to be the problem here?"

Bam-Bam got right to the point. "Fuck off, asshole."

So I said, "Really? Come on, man, you don't want a fight. What good is that going to do? People are just here to have a good time."

"He's too much of a pussy, the big fancy football star coward. Fuck you, Hollywood," he taunted.

"Don't you call me names, shithead." Hollywood was about to clobber the guy.

I interjected again: "Look, sir, if you get into a fight, what's the point, right? We'll have to call the police, you'll get arrested, and then you'll have to call a lawyer. . . . It's Friday night, so you'll probably spend the weekend in jail. Why not just find a way to enjoy the evening?"

"Because the guy's a pussy and I can take him."

"Yeah, we can all see how strong you are. I know you can kick my ass too, but what does that really prove? They only hire me for this job because I'm good looking." I laughed; Bam-Bam did not. "I'm not a tough guy like you. You have to spend a lot of time getting to be that big. I know that and I respect it. Do you really want to ruin your night by getting into a fight right now?" (Hey, I had to give the guy something, and he bought it.)

Henderson was quietly seething throughout this. The guy was so annoying and stupid—and more than a little drunk.

"What's it going to prove?" I continued. "Hollywood is a big, strong guy, and you are too. A fight isn't going to prove anything. But it will get you arrested. So let's just call it a night and go have some fun, right?"

My admission that he could beat me up soothed him. Bam-Bam pumped his chin out toward Hollywood, said, "Fuck you," and turned and walked away. The whole thing was over and I avoided getting myself destroyed in the middle of two very large dudes. Hollywood was grateful. He didn't want trouble either.

Another evening at Confetti's, things didn't go smoothly. Some guy parked his fancy sports car in the "No Stopping" fire zone. The space was clearly marked, with red lines crossing the entire lane and signs posted at either end. Still, this jerk decided to leave his car there.

"Sir, you need to move your car, please," I said with accented courtesy. It had already been a long night for me.

"Fuck you." He was a classy guy.

"Sir, I'm sorry, but this is a fire lane, and you may not park here."

He had arrived drunk. "Leave me the fuck alone! I'll park where I fucking want to, cocksucker!"

"Sir, if you give me your keys, I can move it for you." Given the way he was slurring his words, he shouldn't even have been behind the wheel.

He turned on me then and attacked with a poorly aimed punch to my face. I had at least three inches on him, never mind his impaired faculties. He never should have picked this fight.

I grabbed his outstretched arm and twisted it behind his back, encircling him in a bear hug from behind. His head accidentally slammed into the plate glass of the club, mashing his oily nose against the smooth, hard surface. I held him like that until my fellow bouncers came over to escort him away.

Sometimes you can talk a guy down, and sometimes you must fight back. But sometimes you can't do either. I had had one shivering episode in the first ICU and then another one that landed me in the Atlanta ER. These fits of shaking were so violent that, aside from the general terror that a complete loss of physical control evoked, I was afraid I was going to really hurt myself.

They turned out to be panic and anxiety attacks (P&As) and were not isolated events. They had been occurring since my very first stroke, but it was all chaos in my brain back then. In Nevada, as I began to heal in earnest, we discovered the many layers of my illness.

As a result of my strokes, the chemical functioning of my brain was severely compromised. Every time something weird happened in my brain, which, because of the strokes, was several times a day, my brain would release extra adrenalin: I would have a panic attack. Though not all as bad as the ones that sent me to the Atlanta ER, I would get sweaty, shaky, dizzy, and nauseated. The heightened symptoms would then exacerbate the attack, convincing my brain to release more adrenalin. It was an ascending spiral, and because of this, panic became my near constant companion.

It didn't feel like panic, per se. I just felt like I was dying. My brain was like a herd of elephants on the African plains, grazing peacefully in the blazing sunshine. These elephants, though, were so jittery that they kept stampeding over the slightest, most insignificant offense. They couldn't discern between actual threats and some normal part of nature.

The doctors prescribed Xanax to control my anxiety. But the Xanax also increased my dizziness and light-headedness, making me feel worse than the nerves, so I quit it. Valium also made me feel like crap. I couldn't do it. I preferred to fight my battles myself, even if I had nothing to fight them with.

Sam tried to give me logic as a weapon, telling me my brain was fooling me into believing something bad was going to happen again. "Kevin, these aren't isolated, illogical things that happened. The strokes are due to a *series* of events. The aneurysm built up over a period of time, forming and releasing clots down your arm. The lump was prodded and kneaded, which broke the clots off and made them available." She had my undivided attention, and she was trying so hard to soothe me. "When your neck was twisted, it just created the perfect vacuum to suck the clots out and into the bloodstream going north, into your brain. You are very lucky they didn't go to the places that would have killed you or paralyzed you. The aneurysm was neutralized, there are no more clots, no more neck adjustments, and your arm pain is from residual nerve and tissue damage. This is it. Nothing new here. It's not getting worse, only better from here on out."

I am sad to say that none of Sam's arguments penetrated deeply enough to keep my demons at bay. Logic doesn't work on wanton fear and anxiety. Knowing the explanation did help a small amount, but understanding and trusting that knowledge are two very different things. When all was calm and I was feeling less stressed, I could accept that reasoning for my soaring emotions. Most of the time, though, the P&As eclipsed rational thought, leaving me struggling just to get through the moment. Gruesome speculations about my future tormented me. I was depressed and strung out on drugs that manipulated my emotions and personality. Every new pain, every twinge, each headache made me more paranoid. As I weaned off the blood thinner, I was terrified of more clots forming. It kept me awake at night.

I had been hit by lightning once before, in getting my own TV show—not an easy thing to do in Hollywood. I was struck by lightning again when that show became the most watched TV show in the world, and then again when I landed in the hospital with complaints that were inexplicable and a health crisis that was "one in seventy-five million." Clearly, I was a lightning rod. What could possibly prevent me from being struck again, including by the as-yet unthinkable?

The doctors' prognostications and perceptions about P&As were sketchy, and their drugs ineffective. In due course I learned that time did indeed heal, albeit while I gritted my teeth. Eventually, after more than a year, my brain somehow succeeded in recalibrating its adrenalin-dosing mechanism, and gradually my panic and high anxiety loosened its grip. P&A attacks are not logical. For most of that time I could not persuade, cajole, or convince my brain to calm down and end this. I was just a by-stander, caught in the path of the frantic elephants and torrents of dust.

While I was on my couch every day in Vegas, I was a quiet catastrophe. With no energy and very little distraction, I could fully concentrate on my miserable state. I had the constant sensation of falling backward, physically as well as symbolically. I was as heavy as a boulder, dizzy like a top.

I wish I could say that I didn't feel sorry for myself. What was I supposed to do—think of others? Thinking positive things when your health is absolutely tanking is difficult. You become self-absorbed: *my vanished past, my lost future*. I was clinically depressed, for sure, if that counts as good reason.

I wanted full disclosure. I was angry. I wanted revenge, but on whom? God had tried to warn me. The doctors were simply trying to save me or at least solve my pain. *Hercules* was due to start up again soon (could I even play him anymore?), and who would hire me after the show was finished? My lifestyle was threatened, financially and otherwise; I might never play sports or work out again. I was looking at losing everything, and in my miasma of self-pity and frustration, life looked very bleak.

One late night I was still on the couch after another grueling day, and Sam came to help me upstairs. Gizmoe lay next to me, unmoving. I knew that sleep would not come easily to me, and I was at an extreme low. "You know, Sam, with the way I'm feeling these days, I get it. I really understand why people commit suicide."

Wow. If I was looking for attention . . . Sam knelt down on the floor, facing me, leveling her eyes at me.

"Oh, don't worry. I'm too stubborn for that. I am just saying that all my life, I never understood people who could take their own lives. I looked at it as such a weakness, but now I get it."

"Why are you saying this?" she demanded quietly.

"I don't know. I just realized. I . . . I *get* it. This is really hard. I'm . . . I'm having a really tough time, and I don't see the end, you know? I know I'll get better, but I can't *see* myself better. I'm . . ." I was tired, and this was a painful conversation.

"It will get easier, Kevin. And you are strong enough. You will get better, I promise you." Her voice was fluid and calm as she took my hand.

"I know I will. I just . . . it's like I'm outside the ballpark during the biggest game. I'm alone. *Nobody* understands. Not even the people who know. Not even the doctors who *should* know."

"Yeah. It's hard to keep silent about what's going on, but even if you did come clean, they can't get it—it's too foreign, even if you explain it to them. It's like money, Kevin. Everyone understands a ten-dollar bill, but no one can really wrap their head around a billion dollars—too many zeros. You have kind of like a billion-dollar headache."

"Yeah, 'jackpot.'" I still had my sarcasm intact.

We sat quietly for a few minutes, with Sam caressing my hand and arm. "Kevin, *I* know and *I* understand. And Gizmoe knows too, and she cares. So you aren't entirely alone. Screw the rest of them, right?"

"Yeah. Screw 'em, I guess." She was right—nobody could get it. I recognized my isolation, and there was nothing to do for it. But that didn't make it easier.

As for my suicidal thoughts, thank God I have and always have had a very strong will to live—to succeed, to win, to triumph. But I no longer look upon people who commit suicide as cowardly, selfish individuals. They just need more strength. To never give up. To fight for life. Because whatever ails you, you can survive and beat your demon. One way or another.

You simply have to want life badly enough.

BREATHE

"KEVIN, HOW ARE YOU?" Beverlee's voice sounded subdued and concerned on the phone.

"I'm hanging in there, Bev. What's up?" I was in position on the couch, as usual.

"Well, Kevin, remember the Bengal Boys?"

"Yeah, sure." The Bengal Boys were twins with several degrees of black belts each. Bev represented them in their acting goals. They had wanted to guest star on *Hercules*, and I had tried to get them booked for it, but because they were twins, casting them demanded a very specific scenario.

"Kevin, they heard about what happened to you. They thought they might be able to help you a little bit."

"Bev . . ." I started. I didn't really want to see anyone, and I wasn't about to work out or do any roundhouse kicks.

"Listen, Kevin, some breathing techniques might be helpful for you. Let them come over, give you some tips. It can't hurt. They want to work with you, and they admire you so much."

I sat on the couch, contemplating what this might cost me. Breathing techniques. Beverlee was quiet on the other end of the line. "I appreciate the offer, but I'm just not really . . ."

"Kevin, they are close by right now, in Henderson. Just have them over for a few minutes. It may help you, you never know." She wasn't taking no for an answer. "They are only in town for a few days. Can I give them your address and send them over?"

"I'm just not doing so good, Bev, so they need to understand that."

"Of course, Kevin." I knew she was only trying to help, but I wanted to be left alone; I was such a wreck these days.

Later that afternoon the Bengal Boys, Bob and Bill, stood on the doorstep as Sam opened the door for them. They were smiling, fit, and obviously had abundant energy. I looked at them and thought, *Man, I used to be like that.*

I raised myself off the couch and held on to the top of a bar stool, letting them come to me to shake hands. I vainly attempted to cover up my frailty, but I could see the muted surprise in their eyes. I had lost a lot of muscle mass. We said some friendly hellos and talked for a few minutes about what they were doing in town.

Then Bob spoke frankly: "Kevin, we heard about what happened, and we know you've been through a lot."

I wondered how much they really knew. Bev had been sworn to secrecy, like all of us.

"We think that if we can give you some simple instructions on deep breathing and meditation, it can help you through your recovery and maybe even speed up your healing. Breathing can be very beneficial."

"I know, guys, and I'll give it shot. But I just have to warn you: I'm not what I used to be—not even close." They both nodded in understanding, their hands folded in front of them.

"Let's get to work," Bill proposed quietly, indicating the floor.

They had me lay down on the carpet, on my back. Bill was in charge. "Kevin, I want you to concentrate on a place where you feel happy. Maybe it is a sunny day. Maybe you are outside. Is there a breeze in the air? What does it smell like?" He encouraged me to focus on a specific place, concentrating on the details, and he talked me through a breathing exercise. Guided meditation, it was called. I liked imagining the bright sunshine on a Hawaiian shore, with cool, humid breezes and the smell of the ocean. Although I was on the floor, the world around me was still spinning, distracting me from their instructions. I was like a child in the candy aisle, and my illness was the intolerant parent dragging me out of the store. I tried harder. Anything to get out of the hell I was living.

I felt awful when we were done, in fact, but I figured that was from the exertion of just having visitors as well as from the exercises themselves. Since that day I have resorted to their techniques often. Meditation and controlled breathing can be helpful practices, but both are extremely challenging for an impatient patient like me.

My entire recovery in the desert was a confusing, educational time for both Sam and me. We gradually learned how to handle the curveballs my illness threw, which included some frustrating mysteries.

We went to the movies one evening. Oops. The noise and visual stimulation in the theater messed me up good. Who would think that if I were feeling well enough to get in the car, I couldn't sit in a theater?

Think again, my brain answered.

It took some time for us to understand that the pixel vibrations on a computer screen were causing some of my headaches, dizziness, and nausea. Sam searched for a computer with a different type of screen, but she couldn't find one.

After we realized I could not look at a computer screen, Sam thought that I might have a problem with fluorescent lights for the same reason. The screens and the lights both operate at lower frequencies than incandescent bulbs. My brain was so sensitive that even imperceptible flickering had a negative impact on me. Grocery stores made me feel worse, along with the newer churches in Henderson. When we went to a doctor's appointment, Sam would automatically shut off the lights if there was a window. How much less normal could I get?

I found out the answer to that question much later. Over a year into my recovery Sam and I were visiting with friends on Long Island. It was a beautiful autumn afternoon, and I was having a good day. I was outside enjoying the air with Gizmoe, who was looking for deer to chase.

Coming in hungry from the December chill, I saw a bag of chips on the kitchen counter, so I grabbed a few and ate them while I scoured the fridge for some real food. My symptoms hit me like an invisible wrecking ball: a double dose of dizziness and a splitting headache. Sam walked in smiling, asking, "So are we having venison for dinner?"

I looked at her, frantic I was having another stroke. I said, "I don't feel well. My head is killing me. It just came out of the blue. I need to go lie down." It was so frustrating that my illness had me on this invisible leash, making me heel, making me lie down, making me roll over.

"What happened?" Sam was always so methodical that she immediately launched an investigation, but I wasn't interested. Frankly, her analytical tact annoyed me.

"Nothing 'happened,' Sam. I was fine, you know, feeling pretty okay. I came inside for some food. I just ate a few chips, and it hit me like a ton of bricks, for no reason." What was she going to say to that? Nothing, I figured. But she surprised me.

"Chips?" She seized the package. "Oh my gosh . . . it's MSG, I bet. You're allergic to MSG." She looked surprised at the words that had just come out of her mouth.

"How can that be? I've never had any problem with it before now."

She answered quickly, shaking her head. "You can't possibly know that. You've been sick for over a year, with your symptoms coming and going with no rhyme or reason. Maybe an MSG allergy, brought on by the injury, has been intensifying your issues all this time—and you never knew. Oh, my goodness, I've been cooking with it all this time. It's in every can of soup! I've been feeding it to you!" Her hand went to her mouth.

Believe it or not, she turned out to be right. We did a few experiments, and I definitely had a strong sensitivity to MSG—monosodium glutamate—an additive that is basically used in everything that tastes good. Much of the food we ate was laced with the stuff.

The food sensitivity symptoms mimicked my brain issues. In all fairness, my stroke symptoms were totally across the board: There was really no way to know what else might also be causing similar problems, but nobody had anticipated this aftereffect of my head injury.

A friend suggested that just being in the supermarket could also trigger the MSG reaction, especially down the chip aisle. I never knew for sure; I had stopped going to the grocery store because of the lighting.

But after that, when I got a massive headache after eating, we inevitably discovered that the food had MSG in it.

This new restriction was salt in the wound (pardon the pun), even as it set me free from some of my headaches. What? No more Doritos? Damn, that's harsh!

But it did help me feel a little better as well as vindicated for my reactions to the drugs the doctors had prescribed. Clearly, my brain and illness didn't play by the rules that presumably applied so generally to others, but a new allergy established that I wasn't hallucinating those results: My brain chemistry had obviously changed.

One of the most difficult lessons I learned from my illness was that *resting* is actually something one *does*. I was forced to spend countless hours on the couch, doing "nothing." I thought about all my time spent rushing, sometimes not even knowing where, understanding only that I would know it when I got there. I wondered about where my hurrying had gotten me: sitting on a couch, waiting for healing. I had been the protagonist of my entire life, the dreamer of dreams. Now, my dream was simply survival, and the hero . . . well, it wasn't the queasy guy on the couch.

My meditation carried me to God's feet. This arrival wasn't so much a choice as a result of my mind walking a path that always led me to something greater than me. While I was growing up, Pastor Nordling shouted down hellfire and eternal flames of misery on us sinners every Sunday. He was a scary guy for a little kid, but I recognized manipulation when I saw it. Rather than being frightened into submission, I rejected his teachings, and I rejected him.

Even as a young boy I was able to differentiate between the church and the God who founded it. I was young, opinionated, and logical. I remember asking my mom when I was around twelve years old if God was really *that* mad at us—because I didn't think so. If God could be so evil, why serve Him? He gave us free will. That is a formula for both good and bad things to happen. I thought that, if anything, God was probably sad a lot of the time—sad for the destructive choices so many of His children make. I regarded our pastor as a messenger who had somehow gotten his message confused. I trusted in a loving, forgiving God. I knew God had tried to warn me about this head thing. I blamed myself for failing to understand, failing to react in time.

Before my illness I was fully preoccupied with the material side of life. Moving at the speed of light, I ignored the spiritual side, the unseen. God created this world, but I was determined to live in it to the fullest, to get the most out of it. I figured He would want that. I believed the saying about not going gently into that good night but instead sliding into your grave sideways, screaming, "Wow! What a ride!"

So much for that plan. Lying on the couch with nothing but spare time, I conversed with God and told Him my problems. I asked His forgiveness—for my stupidity, for not listening, for my stubbornness, even for my wasted anger at people. I had worked so hard to get where I was and yet I still was not satisfied. Before this I always wanted more. Now, I just wanted *different*. I begged Him for some understanding.

I thanked Him for not letting the strokes kill me and for giving me the chance to still be a father.

I asked Him to make me whole again. But if this was the best I was going to ever feel, then I asked God to make me strong enough to handle it—stronger than I was now.

I laid it all out for Him and we had some pretty long talks.

God seemed particularly reserved and didn't answer right away. In my impatience I expanded my search for alternative healers. I saw an acupuncturist in Vegas named Dr. Wong. He was Chinese, and he spoke English very poorly. He stuck a bunch of needles in me, which was unpleasant to say the least. Apparently, I'm one of the very few people who *feels* the needles. I really had become wuss of the year.

Dr. Wong's treatments were not effective enough for me to go back more than five times. But he did leave me with one lasting piece of advice. He said, "You—velly happy?" He held his hand, palm up, in front of his smiling face and then shook his head, frowning, "No good. You—velly, velly sad?" His palm went down low and he frowned directly into my eyes for emphasis while he shook his head back and forth, wagging his finger at me. "No good! Not so happy, not so mad—bettah." His hand, palm down, smoothed an invisible tablecloth in front of me.

Extreme emotion was not good for me, he was saying; I needed to remain even-tempered. Boy, he had that pegged right. The problem was that everything was emotional for me these days. I had always run hot, but now my brain, well, it was like it had a mind of its own. For him to tell me not to get too stimulated was like telling Google not to search. Impossible!

I was furious at the illness because of what it had stolen from me. I was angry at my symptoms for what they did to me each day. My limitations and my suffering constantly stoked my rage and irritation. His prescription for me to calm down, in fact, only added fuel to my fire.

Then he said, "You not make happy too offen, yes?"

I looked at him, stupefied.

"You, mellied . . . make happy wit wife? No good." He put his hands up as if to stop me, scowling like an old nun in a parochial school. "Maybe one time—two time in mons."

Shit. Screw you and the horse you . . . oh, who was I kidding? I knew that sex, or more specifically, orgasm, was an issue for my battle-weary brain. He was only speaking the truth. That he knew such an intimate detail of my failures was embarrassing, but he wasn't wrong.

Perfect, I thought. *With all the crap I'm going through right now, this guy is telling me no more sex!* Not that I was a testosterone animal since my strokes—in fact quite the opposite. For the first time in my life, sex was awful. I mean, it made me feel awful. But I couldn't help resenting Dr. Wong for knowing it.

I learned from Dr. Wong that I needed to find a way to control my overcharged passions, but that wouldn't come for a while yet. I took his comments and filed them somewhere in the back of my head, and every so often I pulled them out, acknowledged them, and then stored them away again.

TO BE OR NOT TO BE

IN OUR ACTING ROLES Sam and I had already been married on *Hercules*, so that was like our dry run. After we first started our courtship the producers booked Sam back on the show for a three-part arc as Serena/The Golden Hind, a half-deer magical beast whose blood could kill a god. Our characters fell in love in the first episode, got married in the second, and in the third Hercules is tricked into killing Serena by his evil stepmother, Hera. Mucho drama.

Sam's six weeks in New Zealand was a fantastic time for our whirlwind romance. We spent most of our time together on set, at the gym, and on dates. I was a lovesick puppy and I only got worse. Luckily, she felt the same about me.

We recited our TV-wedding vows of fidelity and loyalty by a lake at sunset, facing each other and holding hands. Sam wore a beautiful white Grecian gown, and, for once, I got to wear something different from my Hercules yellow chamois vest. Michael stood up for me with the dignity and solemnity befitting a best man. Although it was a fake wedding, the setting was so romantic that it was easy to get caught up in the moment. The scene certainly pitted my romantic heart against my bachelor ego. The ego lost. Less than two months later we were engaged.

Our real wedding seemed more like icing on the cake. Sam had not grown up with fantasies of glorious, Princess Di–type weddings, cutting out photos of dresses from magazines and keeping a list of potential reception halls. Neither of us believed in the pomp and circumstance of the elaborate weddings we had seen. We determined to elope in order to keep things simple.

Garmisch was out of the question, so Sam went online to plan it, settling on Reno, Nevada, which was nearby and had package deals.

That was where people used to go to get quickie divorces, and I was strangely uncomfortable with that choice. After sitting with that idea for a few days I wondered out loud how it might be for my father to see the last of his children getting married so late compared to my siblings.

"You know, Kevin . . . if we elope, your dad can't come, right?" Sam smiled, teasing me.

"I know, I know." I paused, pondering.

"You really want him there? Is it important to you?" A genuine wedding would be different on so many levels. I certainly wanted my dad to come—and the rest of my family too—and Sam picked up on that like a dog with a bone.

"Let's make a list, just for fun, to see how big a wedding it would be. We'll start with immediate family and very close friends only," she said.

"I don't know, Sam. It's a lot of work, and with the way I'm feeling, I don't want a great big thing."

She is a practical, pragmatic woman. She sat down at the small dining table and started writing, beginning with Lynn, my father. Then she asked me for friends' names. I listed the first name that popped in my head, an old friend from high school.

"When was the last time you spoke to him?" she questioned.

As I pictured that last Christmas party—or was it our reunion? Sam jumped into the silence: "If you need to think about it, he isn't close enough."

I have a lot of friends from my youth, friends I've known since preschool. But we wanted to keep the wedding small, so we determined that I would invite only the guys I see regularly. That turned out to be five core people—guys Sam knew too.

Sam, however, had moved around a lot as a kid, so she didn't have lasting friendships from school, having spent her senior year in Sweden.

But she did have a group of girlfriends from Los Angeles that she wanted to invite—five of them.

"What about spouses?" I asked. We thought about privacy but wanted to be reasonable. Sam suggested, "Let's invite spouses, but not dates. We have to invite kids too, and my niece could be flower girl. Hey! Gizmoe can be ring-bearer!" At the mention of her name, the lazy little creature lifted her head off the couch, mildly curious.

"No, wait, Gizmoe will never carry anything down the aisle. We'll make her flower puppy, and Alexis can carry the rings. And let's forget Reno—LA will do, right?"

"Right," I said, smiling.

Our list was twenty-eight people, including us. We figured—incorrectly, as it turned out—that some of them wouldn't come.

In late October, about six weeks into my recovery, my team of doctors recommended a follow-up angiogram and some other tests to verify my progress. I was still on the powerful blood thinners, and the doctors were taking no chances, mainly because the root cause of the aneurysm and the strokes was still unknown. For my part, my symptoms haunted me, and every new pain convinced me that we had missed something. We all hoped further tests would squelch any concerns.

I lay on the cold slab of a test bed with nothing but the flimsy gown and my socks on. The socks were supposed to keep me warm in the sub-freezing temperatures of the operating room, but I was still shivering. I did not relish the tube going up my groin again, but doing an angiogram was the only way to know exactly what was happening with the coils in-side me. What if they didn't clot off but instead migrated down my arm? Or, worse, what if they traveled up into my neck and were busy produc-ing more strokes? That was a distinct possibility, if my relentless brain is-sues were any indication.

"Okay, Mr. Sorbo, here we go. You're going to feel some pressure, maybe a burning sensation." Injecting dye into my arteries would reveal on X-ray all the paths my blood was taking, including if there was still the original or any new aneurysms as well as where the clots were preventing the flow of blood.

The tech's business-like manner did not calm me a bit. He was sitting at his instruments across the room. "Are you comfortable?"

"Not really." I tried a laugh. His life was not on the line.

He said, "Yeah, sorry about that. Here comes the first dose. You'll feel a little burn." It started in my shoulder, radiating down my arm with intense pain and building pressure. I must have winced because he said, "Please keep perfectly still. I'm going to administer another round. Here we go." Again with the fire raging across my shoulder and down. My entire left side felt like it was engulfed in flames; the near-bursting sensation was awful. I closed my eyes, gritted my teeth, and tried to meditate myself away from the moment.

Amazingly, the results of my tests were "awesome." One of the doctors said, "You should start eating more McDonald's. Your arteries are *too clean!*"

Ha, ha, ha. The aneurysm had healed perfectly from the inside! Physically, from the neck down, I was almost as good as new. Only my left arm was compromised by some limited circulation and the resulting nerve and tissue damage. More of those blockages could resolve as the body used other avenues to get the blood flow where it was needed. Lucky for me, the human vascular system has many redundancies.

Weissman ordered an MRI of my neck, seeking to diagnose a condition called Vertebral Artery Dissection. This condition can cause clots simply from a neck twist, such as occur during a chiropractic manipulation. Many people suffer strokes from this each year. Weissman wanted to ascertain the blameworthiness of the neck twist, thus potentially ruling out a secondary clot source. In no position to argue, I submitted to another grueling, pounding, clanging session in a claustrophobic tube.

These are my results:

Normal MR of cervical spine with no evidence of bony abnormality.

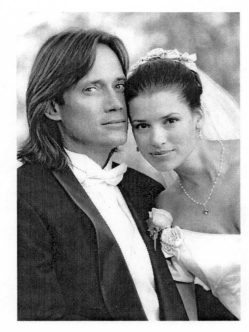

My wedding to Sam Jenkins, four months after my strokes, January 1998. *Photo by Joe Buissink*

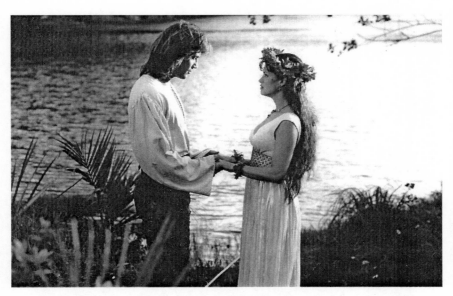

Art imitating life: Hercules marries Serena, December 1996. *Photo shot with my camera; Kevin Sorbo personal collection*

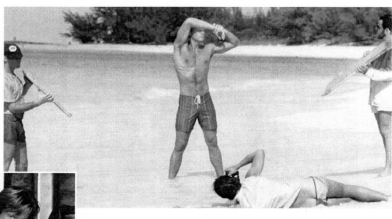

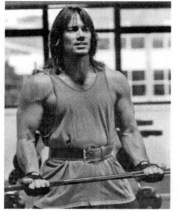

ABOVE: Modeling on the beach in the Bahamas, 1983. *Photo shot with my camera; Kevin Sorbo personal collection*

LEFT: Pumping iron in Auckland just months before the strokes, June 1997. *Photo by Pierre Vinet; Kevin Sorbo personal collection*

Shortly after arriving in Los Angeles, June 1986. *Photo by Kal Yee*

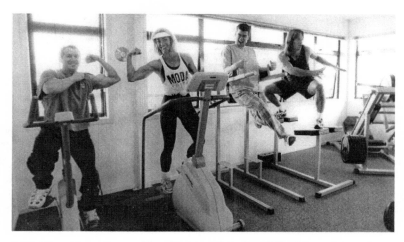

With Steve Rosenbaum, Cory Everson (six-time Miss Olympia), and Eric Gruendemann. *Photo by Pierre Vinet; Kevin Sorbo personal collection*

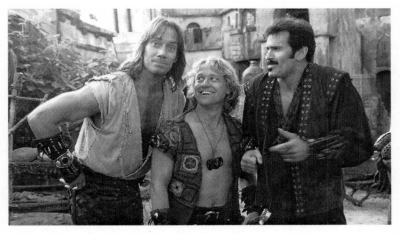

Goofing on the set with Michael Hurst as Iolaus and Bruce Campbell as Autolycus. *Photo shot with my camera; Kevin Sorbo personal collection*

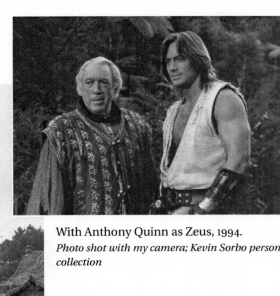

With Anthony Quinn as Zeus, 1994.
Photo shot with my camera; Kevin Sorbo personal collection

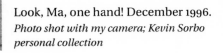

Look, Ma, one hand! December 1996.
Photo shot with my camera; Kevin Sorbo personal collection

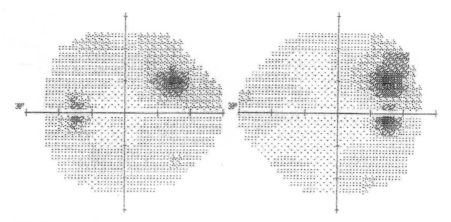

This is a map of my vision after the strokes. The dark spots represent vision loss, September 1997.

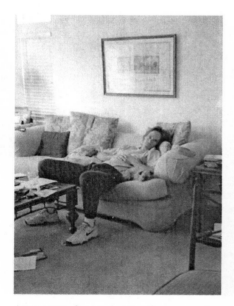

At my townhouse in Henderson, only weeks after the strokes. I wasn't doing too good, October 1997. *Photo by Sam Sorbo*

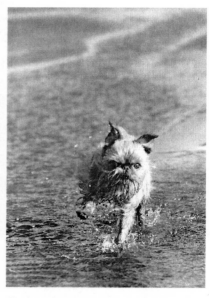

Giz loved running on sand. *Photo by Sam Sorbo*

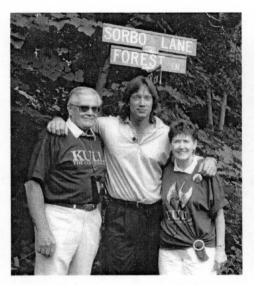

With Mom and Dad by the new Sorbo Lane sign, August 1997. *Photo by Diana Watters*

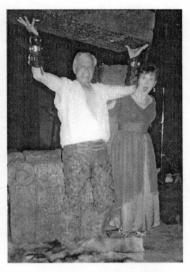

Mom and Dad muscling in on my turf, March 1996. *Photo by Kevin Sorbo*

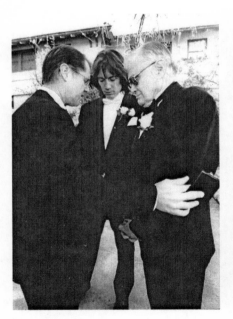

Dad, Pastor Mark, and me praying before my wedding. *Photo by Joe Buissink*

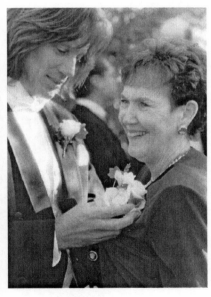

Mom at my wedding. *Photo by Joe Buissink*

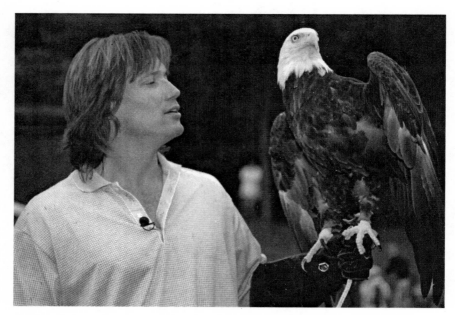

Posing with the University of Minnesota Raptor Center's tame eagle after releasing the rehabilitated one, 1997. *Photo by Diana Watters*

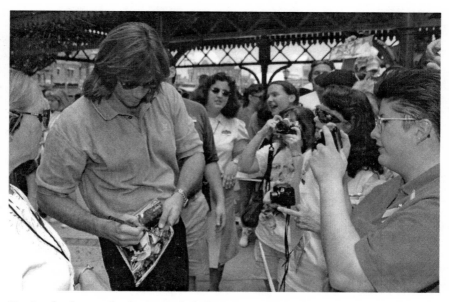

Signing for fans at the Sorbo Park dedication, a week before getting sick, August 1997. *Photo by Diana Watters*

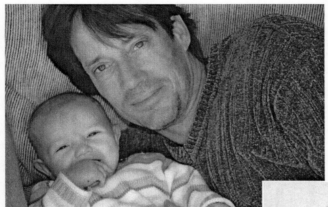

Me with Shane Haaken, my 12½-pound beast, Vancouver, 2004. *Photo by Sam Sorbo*

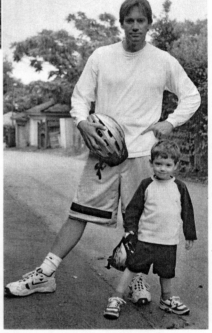

Dad and Braeden gear up for a bike ride, Vancouver, 2003. *Photo by Sam Sorbo*

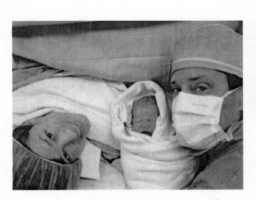

Sam and me with our little girl, Octavia Flynn. The prophecy fulfilled, Henderson, Nevada, 2005. *Photo by Kevin Sorbo*

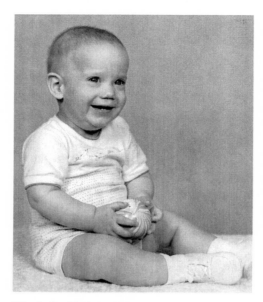

Wee baby Kevin. *Photo by Brenner Studio*

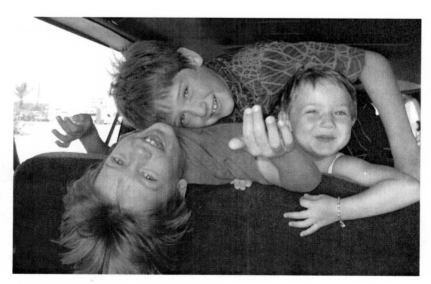

Three little miracles. *Photo by Sam Sorbo*

There it was, in plain print. Fortunately, I did not have this congenital condition, but the results opened up an entirely new Pandora's Box of doubt. What else could have caused my strokes that was unconnected to the aneurysm or neck adjustment?

At least half my doctors doubted that the chiropractic move itself could have produced the strokes, even when combined with a shoulder full of blood clots. *Clots don't swim upstream,* was their mantra. They postulated another explanation for the strokes—a clot source we hadn't found yet (cancer, for instance).

My MRI results continued with this:

Incidentally noted small hypodensity compatible with infarct in left cerebellum.

Translation: Oh, and by the way, there's a little stroke there in your brain, son, which we happened to notice.

Yeah, I know. I have two others up there too, out of frame.

Recent studies have conclusively proven a phenomenon called transient retrograde flow, "TRF," which occurs when severe blockages downstream combine with the right catalyst (i.e., intense pressure or a strong muscle contraction). In this scenario the blood actually surges *backward.* I had hundreds of clots down my arm—log jams throughout. Because transient retrograde flow was virtually unheard of at the time—in fact, it is still a disputed phenomenon—it was not then considered as a possible cause of the strokes.

Years later, when a physician told me about "TRF," I learned that my arm, as full of clots as it was, might have been able to send clots up to my brain with just a bicep squeeze. My third stroke, the speech one, might have been from simple "TRF"—like the final warning shot before a full-scale assault. Doing a push up, hailing a cab, or picking up a bag of groceries theoretically could have killed me. At the time I had no idea how close I had been to the fatal blow.

For the time being, however, we still had no firm explanation for *how* or *why.*

THE SHADOW KNOWS

A FULL EIGHT WEEKS AFTER my initial health crisis, I was not seeing any appreciable improvement. I felt dejected and forgotten. The world was still spinning and people were still living their lives, but for me, time had stalled.

Gizmoe sprawled beside me (as much as an eight-pound dog can sprawl), snoring deceptively. She could be up in a flash, given a suitable incentive. Like Gizmoe, I was waiting for the right catalyst to jump-start my existence.

The phone rang and Sam answered it, as usual—I seldom expended the intense effort to get up from the couch. Sam walked over with the phone in hand. "It's Ned Nalle," she whispered. Ned was an executive from Universal, the studio that owned *Hercules*, and I liked him well enough. A tall, red-headed guy, he always dressed in suits. He was un-complicated and dealt straight with me.

"Hey, Ned, what's up?" I forced myself to sit up, hoping to sound up-beat and casual. Fresh wooziness poured over me like warm mud.

"I'm just calling to check in. We're gearing up to start up production again in two weeks, so . . ."

"Yeah, I know. I'm okay, you know, but it's going slowly."

"I know, Kevin, I know. You know, your health is the most important thing. You have to take care of that or there is no show."

"That's what they keep telling me, Ned." Gizmoe looked up at me, ready for anything. She snorted, making me smile—and wince. I closed my eyes to the bright sun streaming in the window.

"Kevin, they are going to write you very light for when you come back. You can talk to Eric about that in more detail," he continued.

"Yeah, okay."

"You okay?"

"Yeah . . . this is a tough one, Ned."

"You're Hercules, man! You can do anything."

Ned's tone was starting to grate on my headache. I did not like being "handled." I cut in, "I've talked to Eric. I know they're scrambling, but I'm, uh, the doc just said it would take the time it takes. I'm doing all I can, trust me." My hand went up to cover my eyes, not only for the light but also to hold in my frustration. *Of course I want to be back.* I grimaced with the acrid taste of nausea in my mouth. I felt utterly useless. I wanted to scream, thrash out, punch walls, and break things, but I knew any outburst would earn me extra time on the couch.

"I just wanted you to know we are pulling for you, and we are really looking forward to getting you back, big guy."

"Okay, Ned. Thanks for calling." *Please let me get off the damn phone.*

"You bet. I'll talk to you soon."

I laid the phone on the coffee table. Gizmoe was not disappointed when I collapsed back onto the sofa next to her once again. It was just a stroke of luck (pardon the pun) that my crisis had come during a break that was longer than usual to accommodate the film in Atlanta. This allowed me more recovery time than our regular eight-week hiatus would have, but I clearly needed even more.

My illness put a lot of jobs in jeopardy, and it also put a lot of profit at risk. *Hercules* had not yet hit the magic number of one hundred episodes, which the studio needed in order to make a good syndication deal for it. So when executives called, they said things like, "We need to get to a hundred episodes for your back-end deal to kick in—and you know there is a lot of money in it for you in your profit participation." There was a lot of money in it for them too, certainly, but the rest of that story is for another book.

I was desperate to get back to work and pretend that none of this nightmare had happened. I wanted my life back. As much as I disliked the phone calls from the corporate guys and producers encouraging me to get back to work at the end of our hiatus, they spurred me toward my goal. The promise of a great payday was only further incentive.

Besides, what else was I going to do?

Sam had a theory that a person combats any serious illness on three fronts: physical, spiritual, and emotional. I was doing all I could physically to heal my body, and we were going to church and talking with our pastor as well, so spiritually, I was covered. Sam suggested that I see someone for the enormous emotional aspects of my condition. Paradoxically, although that was exactly what I needed, it was the last thing I wanted.

It is a warm October day when I enter the psychiatrist's low-key apartment-office on LA's west side. Sam, who drove, waits in the outer room as Dr. Stutz shuts the door behind me. The room is unimpressive and spare, with a desk much smaller than Stutz's big reputation. It seems he hasn't bought into his own hype. He motions me into a chair near a small card table and takes a seat catty-corner to me.

After I recount what happened to me and where I am now—waiting for ninety days and healing—he answers me in concrete terms, with a New York accent and the swear words to match.

"Okay, this is you." Stutz grabs a sheet of paper and draws two concentric circles, like a thick bubble, around a stick figure. He points to the outer one. "This is you as Superman, I mean the idea—the Hercules you: sleeping four hours a night, going at a hundred miles per hour. The media promoted that grandiose, stylized image."

He draws a few squiggly lines through the outer circle, which reminded me of science class and the sperm fertilizing the egg, and continues, "The strokes shattered that image for you. I know you covered it up for the press, but you still experienced that brokenness. Your secret is

out now, at least to you and Sam. That masculine, hard-charging thing—
you took it too far. You're human—big fuckin' surprise."

Stutz speaks like he is in a hurry to make his point.

I look like Hercules, but inside I am falling apart. *Well, he's got that
much right, for sure, but come on, isn't that obvious?*

"I can't control the neurological stuff, but the He-Man attitude? Uh-
unh." He shakes his head. "The Superman part of you is actually inhu-
man, and you have to fuckin' *abandon* it. That outer shell has to go. You
have to feel deeper than that."

That stops me in my tracks. On some level I probably know that is
true, but do I admit it? *No.* Accept it? *Never.* My goal is for a complete recovery to the heroic, invincible, driven man I have been my whole life.
Here this guy is telling me I shouldn't even *want* that. His words singe
me. I flush, from embarrassment or nerves; his perspective blazes on my
skin and puts a pit in my stomach.

Stutz is in teacher mode, though, oblivious to my raging emotions. Either that or I am a damn good actor. Even in this private session I have
my game face on.

"Now we all have our shadow, the part of us we *don't* want. The ego
wants to leave it behind, but Jung said that the purpose of life is to integrate it—to *integrate* the shadow. You've been denying your shadow for
so long; you've gone as far as you can without it, and now you have to
deal with that. I truly believe you can turn this crisis into progress if you
just get to know your shadow."

I hesitate for a moment. "I feel like I stole something from the five-
and-dime and everyone knows," I say. "I hate it when I'm out in public."

"Yeah, because you feel shame. You were so successful as a Superman-
type, and now you are losing the cloak, and you feel like everyone can
see your secrets. But this will actually take you farther as an actor. You
know those actors who used to be fantastic and then it's like, what the
fuck happened to them? Like they lost whatever it was that made them
so great? Stallone was like that. In his twenties he was actually a really
good actor. Now he just did *Copland.* Did you see it?"

"No."

"Well, you should see it because the character he plays in it, that's his shadow. He fucked around for twenty years denying it, and he was awful. Now he's great again. Jung said that the shadow is the source of flow. The secret of anything intimate is from the shadow."

"I hate that I let it bother me—what people think when they see me."

"Because you identify so closely with your outer shell, without it you are dead. Your fear is that someone will see your weakness."

Stutz is a fascinating man, and he has a bead on me I cannot evade. I briefly wonder how I got here, caught in his crosshairs. On one hand I feel like I can learn a lot from him, but on the other hand I really don't want to. *I don't want to have to.*

The traffic noises waft in the open window. "Saturdays are by far my busiest days. You know why?"

"No."

"I deal with a lot of big fuckin' actors. Saturday mornings, all the movie reports are in, and these guys, they are all terrified, nervous, jittery. Their movie openings define them as human beings. They've gotten so far, and now their shadow is peeking at them from around the corner, and they can't cope.

"But you have to see that this isn't a *setback*. The *problem* would be to never have to face this issue: getting to be fifty and never actually growing up—because that's what the shadow means. Accepting your weaknesses as part of you. There is a priceless benefit to learning this lesson now if you can learn it."

He watches me, I suppose to see if his words are penetrating my hard skull. I shift in my chair before speaking, "I've had a lot of time to think about why. I figured it must be God saying, 'Wake up!' or 'Change your ways.' I mean, I wonder about the doctors who sent me straight back to work."

"Yeah, you can't blame the doctors though. You know why?"

I shake my head. I can certainly blame them. I *should* blame them.

"Because, well, Hollywood is a really fucked up place, no disrespect to the doctors here. But they saw your image, and they wanted to be supportive of that image." He nods at me. "Your body is telling you to take a rest."

But they want me to be Hercules again . . .

It's as if Stutz can read my thoughts. "Listen, Kevin, your success came once you finished constructing your Superman façade. So you feel like they are permanently linked. But that's the bullshit of it. The key now is to change everything. Like the producer on *Hercules*, Rob? You never wanted to ask him for anything because that would be saying, 'I need from you,' and that would be admitting you weren't super-human."

"Yeah, so asking makes me vulnerable." I think about that for a moment. "I used to pray, give thanks, you know? But now I've realized that I was probably more just going through the motions. I really relied on myself for everything."

"Yeah, Superman—he denies God because he's already all-powerful. You can't survive that kind of mindset. You're liable to go back down to New Zealand and, a few weeks in, after they walk on eggshells around you for a while, they're gonna ask you for more time on the set, for you to be the guy you used to be.

"You are going to have to say, 'I can't do that. I need this from you.' You have to talk to your shadow—to the weaker part of you—and, paradoxically, that will keep you safe. You have to do that or else this thing'll fuckin' kill you."

"Okay," I say, resigned. He leans in a shade, holding my gaze.

"It'll kill you dead, Kevin. Trust me."

RELATIONSHIP

Bruce Campbell

KEVIN SORBO IS TALLER THAN ME. It takes a big man to admit that.

This became evident the first time we met on the set of Hercules back in 1994. As a first-time director, my initial goal was just to figure out how to "connect" with the star of this new show.

Thankfully, Kevin, who was very gracious during my freshman effort, broke the ice. "Do you golf?" he asked, in that deep voice of his.

"Heck, yeah, I do," I boasted. Granted, I couldn't golf my way out of a wet paper bag, but what was I gonna do—say no?

"Great," he said with a friendly smile. "Let's go out on Sunday."

I was more than intimidated, but we were off and running. Golf turned out to be a great way to bond. Kevin and I actually had a lot in common: we're similar in age, from the same part of the country (he's a Minnesota guy and I'm from Michigan—both with brutal winters), I had just starred in a male-oriented action show of my own (The Adventures of Brisco County, Jr.), and neither of us liked the baloney side of the film business. The idea of "partying" or "networking" to "get ahead" never made sense to me, mostly because memorizing my lines for the next days' work kept me plenty busy. Kevin seemed like the same kind of guy. As an actor, he was very creative, but he never saw himself as being above the character or the show.

Our first episode went mostly without a hitch, and I counted myself lucky to cut my directing teeth with such an amenable, professional actor. I became more involved in the show as it progressed, sometimes joining Kevin onscreen as Autolycus, the King of Thieves, and we had a blast over six seasons and something like eighteen episodes together.

Naturally, on weekends, when it wasn't raining sideways in Auckland—which happened a lot—we continued to play golf. Sadly, my game didn't improve and Kevin's never got any worse. I would mostly stand in awe of his epic tee shots, shouting "He's Hercules!" if he really tagged one and trying not to lose more than three or four balls each game.

Having acted in some pretty physically demanding roles myself, I appreciated what Kevin had to go through day in and day out on that show. He not only had to look like Hercules, which meant his fair share of time in the gym, he had to perform way more than the average amount of stunts and then charm the beautiful co-star of the week (Sam, don't read that part), all in a jam-packed, twelve-hour day on set. Other actors have had similar challenges, but they never had to pull it off for six years in a row.

As a result of his insane schedule, Kevin was in tip-top shape. That's why watching him endure a life-threatening physical challenge was all the more alarming. I had barely heard of the word "aneurysm," and nobody likes the word "stroke" unless it's associated with golf or swimming, so when word got out that Kevin was sick, I was scared as hell—and it wasn't even happening to me.

Information was very sketchy at first. I assumed that this was because his condition was still being evaluated. Nobody on the production end of things knew what the outcome would be or when he would return— if ever. Obviously, this threw everything into chaos. Kevin was the leading man in the number-one rated syndicated TV show, so there was a lot riding on this man's broad shoulders.

Eventually, the news trickled down. Thankfully, he survived an ordeal that might have killed a less physically fit person, but the questions came fast and furious. Everyone talks about "getting back to normal," but an actor doesn't live a normal life. In their profession they have to shine; they have to look healthy, be intuitive, hit their marks, and endure filming schedules that would make an EMT wince. Assuming that Kevin could—or would even want to—return to this particular gig, how long could he work? Were twelve-hour days a thing of the past? What happens now that he's lost vision and has bouts of vertigo and sound sensitivities? Did it impair his ability to remember lines or perform action scenes? Was he a different guy?

HERCULES AGAIN

THE *Hercules* crew and production staff sent a get-well card signed by everyone, urging me back to work. Many of them wrote, "We miss you!" I missed them too. Props outdid themselves on the card: an antiqued, leather-bound book of several tea-stained "parchment" pages with a nice old-looking *Hercules* coin affixed to the cover. The sentiment was what was important though, and the outpouring of affection and concern touched me deeply.

I got the call from Eric Gruendemann. Was I ready to come back to Auckland and try a limited schedule? Was I up for it?

I didn't know, but I was eager to work again. I welcomed any distraction from sitting around doing nothing.

I boarded the Air New Zealand flight 21 from LAX to Auckland the evening of November 26, 1997. I had a twinge of regret leaving Sam back in LA. It wouldn't be a long trip, so we had decided she should stay behind. She needed the time to plan the wedding and arrange her move, but secretly, I figured after two and half months of nursing me and my battered ego, she needed a break too.

The doctors had told me I would be okay to go back to work now, and although in my heart I knew I wasn't, my ego was uninterested in any compromise. I wanted independence, and that meant I had to go it alone: my feeble, petty rebellion against my shadow, I guess—regretting it even as I quixotically embraced it.

I got back to my house and collapsed on the bed. Everything seemed strange and different to me. I dozed a little. I had flown down a day early to acclimate myself for the jetlag—something I never needed to do before, but now I wondered if I would even be alright to shoot the following day.

Eric called to make sure I was doing okay. He was my friend, but the call was part business too. I took a deep breath and blew it out, slowly and silently, feeling my chest deflate. These days this was my way of coping because it didn't disrupt the fragile balance in my head but still gave me a little relief with something to concentrate on. "Well, Eric, I'm not great. I'm just running on fumes right now. Let's talk in the morning, okay?"

I hung up and sat on my terrace in the back of my rented house, looking out across Lake Pupuke. The humid air and early summer chill made me shudder. The lush lake setting had always calmed me, but now I felt like a stranger.

The scenery was vibrant and green. I was pallid and unsteady. I didn't belong here. What had been so certain before—everything—was now in question. I wondered what I had left to give to a character that I had created and, in so many ways, had equally created me.

The following day my assistant picked me up. We said the perfunctory hellos, but the car ride was abnormally quiet. I had a hard time looking out the window—the speeding images were too much for my compromised brain and my motion-taxed eyes. But when I shut my eyes, nausea hit me full-force.

Annie, in makeup, was excited and happy to see me. She reined in her elation after she hugged me briefly and had me sit in her chair. As Stutz had predicted, everyone walked on shattered glass around me.

When I finally came on set to shoot, I was met with silence. The ever-wry first assistant director, George, put his hand gently on my shoulder and said, quietly, "Welcome back, big guy." Even he was cowed into thoughtful sincerity by my infirmity.

After a brief, awkward moment, I smiled and nodded my thanks.

As he steered me to my seat for the scene and the camera guys jumped in to do final measurements, I looked around at these friends, my coworkers for five years, and I saw love and respect—and also pity. It was just as well I would be sitting for the scene. Their genuine outpouring of support overwhelmed and humbled me.

I was on set for an hour that day. Over the next two weeks I shot scenes for three episodes. Production had transformed the shooting schedule to put me in for as little time as possible each day, but I think they realized they had *overestimated* my abilities. We all had, I guess. I was a complete weakling, forced into submission by my fragile condition. They ordered up more rewrites and new episodes that didn't need me as much.

PROFESSIONAL

George Lyle

Kevin always impressed me with his preparation. He was guaranteed to know his lines, never created a fuss, and knew how to work his way around problems. This kind of commitment (rare in our business) is what gets noticed by the other actors, and it shows the crew that they are dealing with someone who is totally involved. They get behind the star 100 percent. The crew often commented to me about Kevin's focus, and more than one actor told me that they were embarrassed by Kevin's level of readiness. Kevin sometimes even gave his lines to other performers if it made more sense for the scene. This level of professionalism and generosity created a wonderful tone on set that continued until the end.

As a first assistant director on the show, I was in charge of scheduling our shoot days. Eric called an HOD (Head of Department) meeting about Kevin's health crisis, and the cast and crew were told to stay low key. First off, we eliminated Kevin from every shot that we could accomplish with either a body- or stunt-double. Every shot—meaning we approached each script and planned exactly which shots he absolutely needed to be in. I remember Kevin was only going to do about thirty to sixty minutes work a day initially. Of course, this entailed a great deal more effort and forethought than usual, but it was perfectly clear that the

alternative was no show. After such meticulous preparations we organized the shooting to get Kevin on and off set as quickly as possible.
When he came back to set stricken, weak, and uncoordinated as he
was, watching him struggle was difficult.

COMMITMENT

John Mahaffie

I can still remember the terrible sense of astonishment and pain I felt
watching Kevin during his first morning back. Like everyone on the
crew, I was there for him, but we also felt helpless. Just performing the
simplest of filming tasks was a challenge for him.

Eric had imposed severe restrictions on what we were allowed and
not allowed to do with Kevin. In his early days of recovery Kevin was so
weak and unwell that the producers strictly forbid even swinging a
sword while standing still. To save him standing for close-ups we sat him
on a chair chocked up to standing height, preserving his precious physical reserves.

Rob Tapert, my executive producer on *Hercules*, was a smart guy who
readily admitted to lacking a sense of humor, but he knew how to lay out
a story and create a hit show. "I don't get it, but you all must think it's
pretty funny." He might not have understood the jokes that cracked the
rest of us up, but he didn't stand in our way either. I had to admire him
for that.

Shortly after I returned to Auckland and the set, Rob came into my
camper. The camper was nothing to write home about, with a small
table where I would study and an upholstered bench at the back to lie
down on. Drab curtains separated the bunk and driver's cab from the
rest of the small space. There was just enough room to change clothes,
and the color scheme was from a 1960s kitchen. It was cramped quar-

ters, even alone, and with Rob standing in the open doorway it became slightly claustrophobic.

"Kevin, how you doing, big guy?" He had a short, choppy manner of speaking, and thankfully he didn't waste much time on frivolities.

"I'm doing okay, sir. Today's a tough day." They were working on the lighting, and I had about fifteen minutes in my camper before they called me again. I did not want to spend it in idle chatter.

"Yeah, I'm sorry to hear that. I know this has been a difficult time for you, and I just want to say that I really appreciate you coming in and working through it. I mean, we are doing—going to do—everything we can to make this as easy as possible, but we really need to keep the show going. We all stand to make a lot of money on the back end when we finish. You know it all comes down to that."

"Yeah, I do."

Rob and I had had our differences over the years. He was not on set very often, spending a lot of time in the United States. When he was in New Zealand he obviously preferred my show's third-year spin-off *Xena: Warrior Princess* because he was dating its star.

Rob had asked me to write to the Universal Studios executives explaining how important it would be to have a spin-off show that complemented mine, that both shows would benefit from each other over the long run. I agreed, of course.

Once the spin-off was solidly in production, Rob asked me for a list of my favorite directors and writers. They all went to work on *Xena*, and my show never saw them again. I felt betrayed. (It is obvious now that I was *way* too attached to my job, because I took it personally.) After that, I became very guarded around Rob.

This day on set was especially taxing because we were shooting a fight scene. Even though I wasn't really in it, I had to start it and go through a few of the motions so they could cut back to my face at certain points. The head-turns they needed and the few bobs I did to sell that Hercules was actually in the fight wreaked havoc on my brain. (We were still learning my limits, and after that day we would cut my participation down even more.)

Equally as exhausting were all the kinds of emotions that were puls-ing through me: depressed that I couldn't do the fight; embarrassed by my need for a stunt double, a stand-in, and a body double; nervous that I was making an ass of myself; worried that I couldn't even pull *that* off. I kept myself together in front of the crew, but inside I was shaking like a leaf. My efforts would last for only so long and then I'd collapse like a bounce house with the motor off.

I certainly did not want to break down in front of Rob, a source of ag-gravation in his own right. I needed privacy to relax and regroup right now.

"Rob, I really need to shut my eyes for a minute, so if there isn't any-thing important . . ."

"Oh, well, sure. I just want you to know that we're willing to work with you. Whatever you need, we can work it out. There's a lot of money in it if we can get to a hundred episodes—you know that—for you too, Kevin." I was supposed to have the same deal on profit participation as the show's producers.

"Yes, Rob. Thanks for stopping by."

He stepped down and closed the camper door, and I collapsed on the bench.

The truth was that Rob did a lot for me. I recognized that. He had hired me in the first place. He gave the orders to make it as easy for me as possible. He made sure production took care of me, and I thanked him for that. But my symptoms were running my emotions, and "grate-ful" was way at the bottom.

I lay on the bench and wished the dizziness and nausea away. That didn't work, so I turned onto my back and let rough tears wander slowly down the sides of my face.

SCRAMBLING

Eric Gruendemann

AS THE MAIN Hercules producer on location in New Zealand, I was personally involved with Kevin in day-to-day TV-show production, but I also considered him a good friend.

Kevin and I shared several things in common, which had bonded us in a unique way. We were both tall, the only two Americans on the show, and we both had a relentless sarcasm that provided a lot of laughs, the glue we relied on during long days of shooting and short arguments over scripts.

I called Kevin a few times while he was in Vegas recuperating during the show's hiatus. He sounded extremely frail and uncertain, so I was heartbroken for him.

After I spoke with him and gauged his recovery, I saw that he would not be able to shoot his normal schedule. The other producers and I hastily decided to rewrite the upcoming episodes, at least the ones we were shooting before Christmas. Upon managing this tough decision, we realized we needed more time, so the shooting was delayed by at least a week. We even started shooting without him while he was still in Vegas, postponing his limited appearances in the episodes for when he got back down to New Zealand. This, of course, is not the ideal way to shoot any show, but luckily the show was a well-oiled machine at that point, so we managed to get organized enough to pull it off.

We threw out or delayed a bunch of episodes and rewrote more to either write him out completely or have him show up in a very minimal way. I believe we did about six episodes with extremely limited "Kevin involvement" and then gradually phased him back in as he healed and could handle more. Patrick Kake doubled him. We shot lots of scenes over Patrick's shoulder or of Patrick in the distance, and then we might return a few weeks later to shoot Kevin in the scene in close up—anything we could do to get just enough footage of Kevin to put him in the show and then enough footage of Patrick, dressed like Hercules, to maintain Herk's presence in the episode.

We scrambled to eliminate as much shooting of Kevin as possible without needing to rename the show. We did a body-swap episode with Autolycus, "Porkules," in which Herk turns into a pig, and the classic, "Where's Hercules? He's vanished!" kind of thing. We resorted to lots of "Iolaus or Autolycus carrying the show" kind of shows. We did a show about Herk being trapped and needing to be rescued. We did bottle episodes, which use a lot of flashbacks to previous episodes, episodes in which Kevin was healthy. We had to be careful with those, however, because his physique had changed, and we did not want that to be obvious, so we changed the costumes to hide his arms and shoulders.

We jumped every shark in the pond, every last trick we could pull out of our crazy hat.

I am the first to admit that these were not our finest hours, but they got the job done. Along with the schedule pushes, they meant we could keep going overall without totally submerging the series. Our first concern was getting Kevin back to health and not putting that in jeopardy, but the show was in its prime and nobody wanted to lose momentum or cripple us financially by shutting down for months. Having lots of reruns made less sense than original episodes with a minimal Kevin presence. There was a lot riding on continuing the show, so as long as Kevin himself was willing, we were anxious to do what we could for him to keep the show alive.

When he first returned, we literally had him on set for less than an hour a day and for only two or three days a week. This did not include makeup and wardrobe, which took maybe a half-hour. We did have to do some muscle shading and additional makeup to cover for his light wasting and gaunt appearance too.

I specifically remember one episode in which Kevin only appeared sitting on a log. This may have been his very first episode back. He only worked that day for an hour and then we got him home. I was very concerned that we not stress him in any way for fear of doing more damage. I considered that his overall work schedule (our schedule combined with the movies he did during hiatus) had led him to this state of exhaustion, and this may have led to his injury. It was incredibly clear that this man was not the super-human dynamo he had once been; he was very quiet and unsteady. The scene may have been written that Herk was standing, but when he got to set that changed immediately.

The cameras were set and ready to roll. Sound was ready, too, as Kevin walked, tentatively, to the set. Annie, the makeup artist, escorted him. He parked himself on the log, in position, with his elbows on his knees, looking very weak. He had lost a lot of weight and he seemed worried. I knew from our conversations that he was also terrified of having a relapse. I don't think he truly comprehended everything that had happened to him, so he was still processing it. We all were.

The set was very quiet. The normally animated crew was extremely composed, respectful, and efficient. The atmosphere was almost like being at a funeral. I'm not being morbid, just trying to get across how his event had changed everything for everyone on set. We cared about Kevin, and seeing him this way was difficult for us.

"Action!" the director said softly. Hercules straightened his back, trying to look nonchalant, and glanced off-stage at someone approaching. Iolaus walked on set for a brief conversation and then left. Kevin never even stood up.

This was how we convinced the audience that Kevin was still in the show. That hour-long shoot probably got us two scenes, one for the opening and one for the end of an episode. And we gladly settled for that.

QUINN

ON ANY MOVIE SET, the director, along with the first assistant director, who runs the set, usually establish the tone. During the first five *Hercules* movies, we also had the incredibly formidable and forceful presence of Anthony Quinn, who played Zeus, to elevate the status quo. Quinn was a world-renowned actor with two Oscars and two more Academy Award nominations under his belt. He'd done countless films, television shows, and even performed on Broadway opposite Sir Lawrence Olivier. He was, to say the least, intimidating.

I really enjoyed the guy, and I could tell he liked me too. He took to calling me his son (Zeus was the father of Hercules). He was always himself and unflappable, and I learned from watching him.

I also loved the stories he told. The old guard of Hollywood (such as Paul Newman and "Larry" Olivier, as Quinn called him), my inspiration for acting, has all but disappeared now. I got a taste of it during lengthy dinner conversations with this proud, talented icon.

Josh Becker, the young director of our fifth movie (before we went into series), was determined to do a great job, so he came to the set with enthusiasm and an admirable creativity. Early into shooting, Josh meticulously planned a scene between Quinn and me, just how he wanted to shoot it. Everything was ready in the well-crafted barn set, with hay bales and rudimentary tools appropriate for our premise. I would be tying up my horse for the night and Zeus would appear for a father-son chat.

They spent a good amount of time lighting for Josh's shot list (the camera positions for shooting the scene). Although Quinn was not at all a prima donna, a smart director doesn't risk offending his talent; they didn't want to bring in Quinn and then make him wait.

Once he did get to set, the director walked Quinn through all the movement that was to happen during the scene, known as the blocking. "You say this line here, then walk over here and turn toward Kevin. Then Kevin will be here, but go over there and you move away from him, then wait for him to leave. I'll be covering the scene from this angle and then with both cameras from over here." It was a complicated dance— deliberate, like a bumblebee's.

There was one thing Josh didn't plan on. When he finished with his presentation, Quinn, in costume with a fur mantle on his broad shoulders, took a deep breath, turned, and swept regally over to a bale of hay, on which he seated himself with unwavering grace.

"I am going to appear here and stay here the entire scene."

You could have heard a pin drop.

"I . . . am the *king* of the *Gods*," he pronounced in his deep baritone. "I don't move for anyone. I sit, and people come to me." I smiled to myself. *Of course.*

His declaration met with an astounded silence. There was no argument for that. They relit the scene, and from then on Josh deferred to Quinn for blocking every scene he was in.

Quinn did not like to rehearse on set, though he was always eager to prepare scenes in the privacy of his trailer. He memorized his lines, but sometimes they fell short of what his character wanted to express. He theorized that the scene's visuals and its dialogue should tell the story; he was weary of all the exposition.

To solve this problem Quinn would remove any exposition and then make up his own dialogue. His enthusiasm was contagious, though a little frightening. He'd say to me, "I'm going to say something else here, so you'll have to come up with your own answer. You'll think of something, sweetheart." He called everyone sweetheart.

Initially, this was incredibly frustrating and nerve-racking: I am pretty much a "script" kind of guy. But eventually it became fun and made our scenes organic and spontaneous.

I needed some of that spontaneity and *joie de vivre* right about now.

THE WEDDING

Sam and Kevin

"HAVE YOU THOUGHT ABOUT YOUR VOWS?" Pastor Mark spoke softly to Kevin and me in his little office in Eagle Rock. Frankly, there were so many more immediate issues to deal with—our vows were pretty low on the list.

Just over one month into his recovery, Kevin's symptoms seemed to be only getting worse as we discovered his limits. Each time the migraines or nausea would crescendo, I could usually find a trigger to blame. Was I right? I was operating on instinct. I was certain Kevin would recover, but when and how were frustrating questions with no answers. My goal was to give him some peace of mind. I became fortune-teller, cheerleader, comfort giver, and healer to the strongest man I knew. It was an odd twist of fate that I had chosen the most independent, self-motivated, driven person I had ever met—qualities I admired and envied—only to watch him crumble.

"We still need to work on vows. I do know that Gizmoe will be flower puppy. I made her a little gown, with rosettes on the hem." I had sewn it in the recent days while Kevin lay on the couch. I smiled at Mark through glistening eyes.

Mark pretended not to notice my emotions. "Well, these things are pretty straightforward. You might look at the traditional vows and then modify them to suit you. One thing that I've seen couples do—especially

171

with a small wedding—is turn around at the beginning and thank every-one for coming. Tell them what it means to you to have them there."

"Yes! We'll do that too. Kevin?" My upbeat tone sounded forced, even to me.

"Sure, sounds good," Kevin answered quickly. He was having a bad time of it today. Already an impatient individual, his issues taxed him to the breaking point, and my unflagging optimism wasn't helping. I could tell Kevin was antsy to be done here and on the road, heading for the quiet reprieve of the desert.

Mark turned to Kevin, "And how about you, Kevin? Anything special you want me to say or do?"

"Let's just keep it simple," he offered.

"How are you holding up, Kevin? Is there anything at all that I can do for you?"

"Thanks, Mark. Just pray for me, please. Life is really hard right now, and I don't have any answers. Pray for my head to sort all this out and get back to normal, will you?"

"Of course I will. May I pray for you right now?" We both nodded our thanks.

Mark gently placed his hands on our shoulders. "Heavenly Father, I lift up Kevin and Sam to you right now. Father, they are going through such hardship and they need your help. Kevin is hurting so much, and at the same time he is embarking on a new path in his life with Sam. Father, they need your strength and your guidance. I pray that you would send them some comfort and some reassurance, ease their hearts, and bring them some peace. In Jesus' holy name I pray. Amen."

Gizmoe was freshly bathed and fluffy from the blow-dryer; my hair and makeup was finished; and the wedding dress, a simple cream satin gown, was loaded in my car. Kevin wore his tux, waiting for his buddies to pick him up a little later, but I needed to be at the center in Pacific Palisades early to meet the florist and oversee decorations.

The small clapboard-and-beam chapel held only fifty people. It was rustic and romantic with a large wooden cross hanging over a roaring fire in the fireplace up front. My girlfriends were spreading a white cloth on the table where the candles and roses would go, and the florist was on a ladder at the front, hanging a beautiful garland. She had already decorated the front four pews with flowers.

Someone had suggested to me, "Kevin, go into the empty church before the ceremony and sit for a moment in the stillness and solitude." I needed that today, for sure. I thought about my life, what I yet wanted to accomplish, and how insurmountable my injuries seemed. I wanted to change the world and to help people. I wanted accolades like Oscars and Emmys, treasures and fame. I had these desires for greatness. Now all of that faded into the background.

While the driven, selfish, business side of me was steering the ship, a perfect storm had hit, which required someone new to command the boat. I pondered the profundity of the step I was about to take, with sorrow, still, for the deposed captain. I cautiously prayed that someday he would be brought back on deck, but for now we were sailing under new flags and in a completely different direction.

I dedicated the moment to God, thanked Him for saving my arm and my life as well as seeing me to this point. I promised Him I would make a good husband. Never had I needed anyone so desperately before. This was humbling, but I respected the notion that in my need, He had provided. I also asked Him to remove the burden of my affliction once again, not believing that I deserved that great mercy.

I walked back outside and found the pastor talking with my dad. Dad looked fantastic in his dark suit, and he embraced me in trembling arms, a result not only of years on asthma steroids but also, I think, from the excitement of the day. My parents had been happily married for forty-five years, and they wished the same for their children. I wondered if I might ever reach that mark in my marriage.

Being a bride was exciting and nerve-racking. Aside from the pressure of hosting a big party, this was an intensely personal, momentous, and scary step—joining for life with someone, making a vow to him and to God. I could barely contain my emotions.

The violin and cello began Bach's "Jesu: Joy of Man's Desiring." I took a deep breath and my mother's arm, and we started toward the arched doorway of the small church. Two large rose bushes flanked the entry under a small, beamed gable. We strolled through the doorway until, suddenly, my head jerked back. The rest of my body was moving gracefully toward the front of the chapel, but my head would not. (I know—weird symbolism, right? No! Keep reading!)

Unceremoniously, I backed out of the church to see what was wrong. A gust of wind had lifted my long tulle veil, causing it to catch on the rose bush! As I bent toward it, my veil became even more entangled. I handed my mother my bouquet of pale roses and began to try to extricate the gauzy white material. The photographer, Joe, ran out to give a hand. Getting uncaught was not easy.

The lovely music continued. I called out to no one in particular, "I'll be right there!" and heard laughter. Suddenly, the stresses and the pressure that had built up to this moment floated away, like so many butterflies. My entire disposition changed.

I think everyone heaved a little relaxing sigh at the end of the giggles. Joe, Mom, and I carefully snatched the veil back and continued in, joyful and enthusiastic, led by Alexis, my six-year-old niece, and Gizmoe, regal in her handmade gown, greeting each pew with a proud sniff and wagging tail.

Pastor Mark said, "Can I just say, 'Wow!'"

I stood with my dad and Mark as Sam finished the short walk down the aisle. She looked incredible. I knew I was marrying a beautiful woman, but the setting, the music, her statuesque presence—all of it conspired to create an ethereal quality to the moment. I was blown away. "Wow" was an appropriate word.

As we turned to address the filled pews, I choked back tears. "I just wanted to thank you all for coming. It means a great deal to us to have you here to witness our union and our vows. I think Kevin agrees with me."

Because he was so unsteady, Kevin had planned to simply say, "I do" and then make a little joke that he was too early with those words, but he was so emotional that he could barely get out anything. His eyes were brimming, he was shaking, and his lips trembled.

I stumbled through "Yes, thank you so much" and turned back around as the pastor began the ceremony. We lit candles, gave a rose to each mother-in-law, and recited our vows. Pastor Mark concluded with the introduction of Sam and me as husband and wife.

Walking out into the late afternoon sun, I took a deep breath. I had survived my own wedding! We all took photos outside after the ceremony and then headed to dinner at the Four Seasons.

When our car arrived at the hotel, a lot of heads turned. (The event had been booked as the Jenkins' family reunion to avoid any press. I had no idea how I would be managing my symptoms on the day, so the last thing I needed was for my illness to sneak into the limelight again.) The valets, doormen, and front desk and restaurant employees discreetly murmured their devotion to my show and helped out with our guests. The welcome was nice, but I kept a steady pace through the lobby and restaurant to our private dining room. I plastered on a fake smile as my head did whirlies. Once more, I felt exposed.

We enjoyed an animated dinner. Our friends and family are comedic and unguarded, and the Minnesota boys' club meshed nicely with the Hollywood gals. There were toasts with entertaining stories about bride and groom, clinking glasses and glistening dishes, candlelight, rowdy laughter, and heartfelt reminiscing. The background music was soft classical, the food was sophisticated and delicious, and the cake was, well, it was wedding cake. They never taste good, right? We did the perfunctory "cutting of the cake," but not the smashing of it into each other's mouths.

Although I was certain I had chosen the ideal mate, I could not say the same thing for Sam. I knew she loved me, but at the same time I considered the possibility that she was making a big mistake in marrying me. I was a mess, and my prospects did not appear very good either. The idea that I would be burdening Sam with a useless shell of a man weighed on me in the moments when I reflected on our future together, thus amplifying my anxiety. I was already four months in to my three-month recovery, and I still had a very long way to go.

Although the music was low and the dinner noise from the small gathering was minimal, by the end of the evening the generator sound in my head was full throttle. As much as I hated the party to end, it was time to say goodbye to all our friends and family. I was completely drained. But I was happy I was married.

Sam drove us the few blocks to her apartment and helped me down the hall and into the elevator. Gizmoe was waiting excitedly for us at the door, with her little butt wiggling back and forth. I was in no condition to bend down to pet her. I staggered down the hallway, ripping my clothes off as I went. (If only I felt half as sexy as that just sounded.) For Sam and me the wedding night was "untraditional." I needed sleep and rest and quiet and solitude. There would be no marital bliss tonight.

I felt like a failure. What man gets married and fails to consummate the union that night? It wasn't that I was anatomically challenged, of course, nor was it a lack of desire. In fact, my running joke was that I was half-god from the waist down. But my symptoms had hijacked me from the neck up. My head just wasn't in the game.

There would be no honeymoon for us either. After all the scheduling concessions the producers made before the Christmas break, I had to get back to work immediately, and Sam would follow a few days later.

REALITY VS. TV

TODAY IS A BEAUTIFUL SUMMER DAY, January in New Zealand, and the sun shines with the intensity that only a loving deity or a failing ozone layer could produce. The mild humidity provides a pleasant weight to the air. Birds sing, cicadas create that irritating noise we have all grown to ignore, and the set of *Hercules: The Legendary Journeys*, the most watched TV show in the world, functions like clockwork. *Hercules* proposes a world where ancient Greece is combined with modern elements, breaking all the rules and offering a lot of tongue-in-cheek humor. We spoofed on everything from McDonald's golden arches to Hercules inventing bowling and golf.

The scene today begins as Iolaus and I emerge from some bushes, having just dispatched several bad guys in a typical *Hercules*-style fight the fans will love. Prior to my illness, of course, I would have filmed at the center of the entire fight scene in one straight take. The stunt guys are that good. With excellent timing, they always come in on cue to flip, stagger, or collapse suitably and convincingly enough to sell my no-contact hits or kicks.

I used to learn the fights like a kind of dance: duck here, punch there, turn and kick, step back, turn, punch, and jump high. The stunt coordinator, Peter, is a gifted man who loves to throw the unusual or unexpected into his fights. We would often have interesting props to use: buckets, poles, furniture—scene dressing until the fight began. Iolaus and I would exchange taunts, encouragement, or even criticism, which completed the illusion of a world in which I could easily toss a full-grown man through a wall and he would leave a life-sized cut-out of himself for the audience to peek through.

Now, unable to perform the fight scenes even somewhat credibly, I am sidelined during shooting. I get to pick up the action after the action is done.

"Action!" the director yells from behind the monitor. Twenty yards away, the crew has established a "media village," complete with monitors and seating for the director, sound guys, continuity, and other people who need to watch the screens to do their work.

Iolaus and I step out of the lush island greenery. The cameras are a few feet away.

"Wow, Herk, you really could have left a few for me," Iolaus teases, wiping his hands together.

"What can I say? I love what I do."

Except that today I am not loving it. Some days were manageable and others were, well, today is one of those other days. My head distracts me and my footing feels unsure, even on the hard-packed soil. I worry about tripping on the twigs my blind spot conceals.

Michael says his next line: "Just leave some for me next time, okay, Herk?" The scene has all the irony it can hold. He pats my shoulder and almost imperceptibly pushes me, urging me to walk out of the scene, just as we blocked it.

"Yeah, sure, buddy. You got it." I take the three steps I know clear me from camera and then rest my hand on his shoulder, hoping he will stand still for me. I'm a ship swaying in invisible waves. I usually pretend that I am fine, which then exhausts me so much that I collapse when I get back to my trailer, but today I cannot even play-act.

Michael is a good friend and I admire him tremendously. He is a trained Shakespearean actor with the memory of a computer, and he is very good in the action sequences we have on the show.

I remember one of the first fight scenes we had against each other. The show was launching the character of Xena at the end of season two.

(There was no "warrior princess" spin-off yet.) In this introductory episode evil Xena seduces Iolaus and turns him against Hercules. We would have a wicked sword fight.

Michael was theatrically trained to handle all kinds of weaponry, so naturally he insisted on doing his own fight scenes. I was good with that.

During the fight there was this one very dangerous move: With my back to Iolaus, I was supposed to spin down low to the ground. Michael was to swing the sword at where my head would be if I were standing.

I pulled Peter and Michael to the side. "Michael," I said quietly, "Aim high. That last rehearsal you brushed the top of my head with the sword."

"No worries, mate," he replied enthusiastically. "I am the New Zealand fencing champion!"

Well, not today, he wasn't. The fight scene Peter had set up was huge. It began with several parries and big moves back and forth, before Michael's huge sword would sweep over my head. We were both intensely focused on creating the appropriate drama for a fight of this magnitude. When the time came I ducked lower than before (just in case, I reasoned), but Michael swung so low that he nailed me on the back of my scalp. I went down hard; knocked out cold.

When I came to a short time later, John Mahaffie, our DP, was holding me in his arms. I immediately tried to sit up. "Whoa, mate!" John said firmly. "You are looking very pale and you are bleeding pretty badly. We have an ambulance on the way."

The ambulance rushed me to the hospital, where they took some pictures of my noggin to check for internal damage. I had suffered a concussion, and the four-inch gash on the back of my head took all of seventeen stitches.

After viewing the fight scene in the dailies, I realized I was very lucky that Michael had shifted the sword and hit me broadsided, with the flat part of the sword instead of the blade. Although the swords are props, they are not plastic but rather a lightweight metal. With enough force behind them, they slice without difficulty. One can always speculate, but I do believe that if he had hit me with the blade of the sword, I would not be writing this story!

The following day Peter got stunt guys to finish shooting the fight with each of us, and Michael and I never had to sword fight against each other again, thankfully.

Michael was extremely embarrassed and apologetic, and he gave me a very high-end bottle of scotch to patch up our friendship. I didn't sweat him about it. We all make mistakes. I couldn't fault him for being too enthusiastic. Particularly after that incident, Michael and I became much closer.

Today, during my grueling internal battle, he is being the good friend I need, supporting me surreptitiously. I don't have to say anything to him about it; he is just there for me. He can see that I am not the capable guy I used to be, so he fills in where he perceives a need. And I need him more than I would like to admit.

The saddest thing for me today is looking at him looking at me. Michael's eyes harbor a pity that is impossible to ignore, but it is even harder to accept. During the scene, while he is praising my fighting prowess, his eyes ask me if I can make it. *Steady, now? Do you remember your next line? Are you okay to walk now?*

I tolerate his pity only because I have no weapon against it. I understand that it represents the honest reality, not the fantasy world of an implausible, laughable TV show.

ACTION HERO

Michael Hurst

KEVIN WAS AN ACTION HERO. We both were, I guess, but his athletic frame and physical prowess easily allowed him to fill the role of Hercules, demigod and protector of mankind. This, combined with the attention lavished upon the stars of a successful television show, lends the role of hero a certain dominance in real life. I remember Kevin telling me that it was easy to feel invincible—to believe that nothing could go wrong and that all steps ahead were strong and sure.

I was really shocked when he got sick.

I remember visiting him in LA during his recovery. He sat in a darkened room and spoke in quiet tones. His energy was extremely low, and for long periods he would simply sit and stare into nothing. To see this lion of a man so subdued was really quite upsetting. He was dealing with his mortality, he told me, and I think many issues were coming up for him apart from his actual physical well-being. He told me all about what had happened, and he shared his feelings of anxiety and his sense of being lost, of not knowing for sure what the future was going to bring. I remember him saying that he was really concentrating on being in the here and now. I'm not sure if he remembers the visit—we didn't speak about it again—but it had a profound effect on me.

I left LA to return to New Zealand and begin shooting episodes of Hercules that did not, in fact, have Hercules in them. The first one was

"Yes, Virginia, There Is a Hercules," in which we all played the writers of the show who were freaked out because Kevin Sorbo had gone missing. As it happens, this was a major creative sidestep for the show and proved to be very funny and very successful. "Porkules" was to follow, in which Hercules had been turned into a pig (played by a pig) and so required Kevin to actually participate very little.

Kevin returned to shoot only one line for "Yes, Virginia . . ." before slowly easing his way back into shooting. I will never forget the day he came on set. We were told that he would be with us for only thirty minutes and that we had to achieve the shot in that time. We were to avoid rapid movements and loud noises, and we were to keep conversation to a minimum. Lighting was to be muted, and a stand-in had to do everything right up until Kevin stepped in.

I was back with the group, in the shot but with my back to the camera. Kevin came in wearing a suit (he was playing himself for the shot), and seeing how thin he had become was a shock. His face was gaunt and he was moving quite slowly. He was clearly nervous about this moment and was, I could tell, fighting to control his energy. He had to say something like "I'm back" and then wink at the camera. We watched in silence as he said his line in a light voice and then mustered that "hero" look for the camera. I felt the tears spring to my eyes. This was my great big friend—Hercules, Kevin—the man I laughed so much with, the man I really respected and loved, a generous and thoughtful actor who totally loved what he was doing. This was he and he looked so frail and brave.

There was a pause after he said the line and the director called cut. Then George, the first assistant director, quietly said, "It's good to have you back, Kevin."

The place erupted in applause and I looked around, crying, to see others crying too. It was a really powerful moment.

Kevin began slowly adding shooting time to his daily routine, and we got more and more of him in the episodes—first one hour, then two, then four, and so on. But the stunt and doubles departments had to really step up, making sure that he didn't take on too much too soon, and his calls were never too early in the day or too late at night. Often I would begin a scene with the double in the morning and then Kevin would arrive and we would do his shots. Likewise, at the end of the day Kevin would go and I would finish up. This was absolutely fine by me— I was grateful to have my buddy back, and the show just couldn't have happened without him.

Kevin and I talked about this time later, with him remarking on just how very small he felt when the "invincible" bubble burst. It changed his outlook forever, I think. Having said that, we both still went on to have tremendous fun with the show, and once he regained his strength and recovered that sense of hero, he was unstoppable.

There is a photo of us both sitting side by side on set. It was taken around this time. We had had a long day, I was tired, and Kevin was approaching that time when he just needed to go home. He and I are almost the same age and we both came to the show in our mid-thirties. I think you could say that we grew up during the seven years we worked together. We had life-changing experiences and Kevin had a brush with death. Neither of us was going to be the same. You can see that in our faces: heroes with history, I guess.

ROUTINE

My new zealand rented house on Lake Pupuke had spectacular views, but it was, in a word, *weird*. The main room was lodge-like, with a high, beamed ceiling—the unfinished underside of the roof. The master bathroom did not have a door. The powder room had a two-way mirror window that, when the light was on, offered a full show to anyone in the kitchen. And the house had a portion of corrugated plastic roof that resonated with each raindrop, creating a deafening noise that permeated throughout the open floor plan. And this being Auckland, it rained almost every day.

Nowadays I would come home from an hour or two on set, lie on the couch for a while, and then get up and struggle through ball exercises with Sam. At first Sam was not very good at throwing a ball, but this turned out to be the least of my problems! They were incredibly tedious: Close one eye and catch the ball with one hand, then the other. Stand on one foot and toss the ball with one hand, then the other. Yet these exercises were all I had to cling to.

The local boat club used the lake for crewing exercises and races throughout the summer. Beginning at seven in the morning, an air horn reverberated around all corners of the large lake. For lack of anything else I could do, Sam and I would drink fruit smoothies on the back deck and watch the rowers. Saturday mornings used to be my time to catch up on e-mails, script editing, and phone calls—and golf, of course—but those days were gone.

The annoying guy with the megaphone, a surly-sounding type in a boat on the lake, would often reprimand the young crews: "Boat number eight, get back in line please!" "Boat number six, you are facing the wrong way." (I might be making that one up.) Then the horn would blast and the boats would take off. Sam and I joked to each other that it would be great to someday go out there and blast an air horn just to mess with them. We never did it, but we wanted to!

Our suburb, Takapuna, claimed the ocean beach as its highlight. Sam and I would walk over to the beach and then along its shore for an hour. There is something soothing about the waves massaging the shoreline and the cool breezes in my hair. I would breathe in the salt wind and say prayers to the God who created it, willing Him to heal me. I would visualize my heart pumping solid and strong, with the oxygen coursing through my body, feeding my organs and healing me, and this helped me encourage myself to push through the pain, to endure.

On these walks Gizmoe was a happy companion. The beach and the wind was her favorite environment, and she would joyously prance around, chasing seagulls and barking at the waves even as she ran from them.

One afternoon the suggestion of a walk excited Gizmoe so much that we could not get out the door fast enough. By the time we reached the shore, a strong wind had come up, which energized the puppy. Sam let her off the leash, and we laughed, watching her cavort by the waves and basically go crazy in the sand. She loved the sand on her paws, and she ran back and forth, doing whirlies and kicking up dust. When a seagull flew overhead, we watched in fascination. The birds liked to tease Gizmoe; we had seen it before. Gizmoe tore after this one, head high, barking, as she sprinted like a miniature gazelle across the beach.

As fast as that, she was gone, down the beach and out of hearing. Gizmoe was a well-trained dog, but once she got out of earshot, well . . . Sam looked worried, and I could understand why. She said, urgently, "I've got to run down there."

"Go!" I answered, "I certainly can't." She jogged down the beach.

I waited, quietly breathing in the salty wind and resting my eyes on the fading eastern horizon. Eventually Sam made her way back down the shoreline holding a soggy, sandy, utterly exhilarated little furball.

We moved to Remuera, a different suburb of Auckland. Our new rental was a rambling old house with lots of rooms, much more comfortable than the last one. It had good light, nicely painted walls, and no two-way mirrors in the toilets! It had an unheated swimming pool that never crested 68 degrees (those Kiwis are no sissies), and it also had a small, intimate room with no windows and three doors. My comfy white couches fit perfectly into that space, leaving room for nothing else. I describe this room because this is where I spent *a lot* of time. Lying on the couch, watching *The Simpsons*, *Mad About You*, and *Friends* before, during, and/or after dinner.

This was where I retreated to wait for my brain to get better, will it to heal, every day, when I wasn't on set. Sitcoms were an ideal distraction.

This den was also where I would discover Sam reading at three in the morning. Because I woke so often during the night, I would immediately notice the emptiness of the space if she had gotten up. She was a voracious reader, and although she would rather have been sleeping, she never complained about her insomnia that was brought on, no doubt, by worry. She simply read, quietly sipping a cup of chamomile tea.

We settled into a routine. I got up each morning and had oatmeal. I went to work, struggled through my scenes, and fought the headaches, dizziness, nausea, and the humming at the base of my skull. I considered myself somewhat lucky just to keep my day job.

Hercules producers had hired a new young writing team of Alex Kurtsman and Roberto Orci to spearhead the script development for the show. They had original ideas and a creative approach, and I credit them a lot for keeping the show going when I could barely swing a sword. They went on to become a favored Hollywood writing team, turning out *Alias, Fringe*, and *Hawaii 5-0* for television as well as *Transformers*, the most recent *Star Trek* movie, and *Cowboys and Aliens* on the big screen. *Hercules* proved to be a great launching pad for people on both sides of the camera.

The *Hercules* production offered me a gym membership at a new, small, private gym in Auckland. Steve Rosenbaum was the proprietor and trainer.

Initially, I was skeptical about his methods. I had worked out my own way for years and I thought, *why fix something that isn't broken?* That didn't last long, though. Steve revamped my routine, streamlining it in ways I had not thought possible. But the real proof was in my improved physicality.

Steve is in phenomenal shape. He had won awards for an extremely fit and powerful physique, even at fifty. I remember going to see *Titanic* with a small group of people. Steve sat through the entire three-hour movie straight as a rod, with his back never touching the backrest of his seat.

Returning to Auckland a broken and discouraged man, I went to the gym and told Steve everything that had happened. I knew him well enough by now to have confidence that he would respect my privacy, and I needed him to understand how sick I really was.

He listened with honest concern and then said, "Wow, buddy, you've really been through a lot. You've lost a lot of weight and muscle mass, but we can get that back. We'll start slowly and ease you back into it. And with the dizziness, well, we'll stay on the machines for now. Let's get started with some cardio." We both understood that my key problems lay in my brain, not my muscles.

I started each session with fifteen minutes of cardio on the stair-stepper or elliptical. Steve supervised me when I did arms and shoulders, back and chest, or legs. He taught me more effective lifting strategies to get a better workout in less time: low reps with high weights, to exhaustion. He insisted on copious amounts of water—calling it "life giving"—and advocated plain rice and boiled chicken breasts for dinner. He harped on how sugar was "the enemy!" With his positive, gentle encouragement, Steve became a kind of lifeline for me.

I worked out at his gym three times per week instead of my usual daily schedule. Sam would often meet me at Steve's to keep me company and give me moral support, but she worked out as well. Workouts had always been my therapy; now they took on a new significance. Although they were never an escape from my incessant symptoms, the physical workouts with Steve offered distraction and fed my exercise habit. I looked forward to the calm of Steve's place and the intensity that lifting demanded. Soon I saw and felt results; far from just the physical progress, my workouts drastically improved my morale. The exercise gave me purpose, and my muscles' physical exhaustion made me feel somewhat normal again. I was back in control of a small part of my world, for which I was eternally grateful.

After our workouts Sam and I would inevitably head home to dinner on the couch and TV. The schedule was simple: Work came first, then exercise, then lots of rest. (The third part was what had been lacking before I got sick, and now I was making up for that in spades.) It wasn't the fun it used to be, but it was the best I could hope for. My confidence had been shattered, and this uncomplicated routine gently helped me start to regain my footing.

On nongym days Sam and I walked Gizmoe to nearby Cornwall Park. I couldn't jog yet—I was still too dizzy to trust myself not to fall.

At one point in recent history New Zealand had about twenty sheep for every human, so you might imagine that sheep are not entirely hidden out in the boondocks somewhere. Yep, the laws in New Zealand allow sheep and cows to share the city parks with people. And yep, there are plenty of places in the expansive grassy park where you must watch your step. It had that quaint, country vibe, and our walks were both invigorating and relaxing. Even in a light rain, the walk was a destressor and a time for us to just be together.

At the center of the park, One Tree Hill, a 550-foot volcanic peak juts up abruptly from level ground. This site inspired U2's big hit of the same name. Not surprisingly, there is one isolated, craggy tree at the very top, and next to it towers a narrow stone obelisk marking the grave of the park's patron, Sir John Logan Campbell.

The peak, with its two standouts, provides a striking silhouette from below. The memorial was built to commemorate Campbell's admiration for the Maori people, and consequently, for somewhat obscure reasons, Maori have vandalized and attacked the tree many times over the years.

Sam, Gizmoe, and I would habitually ascend the narrow, circuitous path to enjoy the expansive view from the summit. I always took a moment to consider the old weathered, beleaguered tree. It had scars on the trunk, a tattered chain link fence around it, and tethers to hold it in place. It looked like I felt during that period in my life.

But it persevered—and so did I.

KRYPTONITE

Sam and I pick up friends Kevin Smith and Geoff Dolan. We're on our way to Ericson Stadium, a large concert venue not far from Auckland. My set security guy, Jason, whose company also works security at the concert venue, scored us awesome tickets to the Billy Joel/Elton John concert. I've managed my illness and seen mild improvement over the past several months, but more importantly, I'm desperate to be normal again. I'm excited to be going out for the first time since getting sick.

I think I've been to over three hundred concerts in my life. I've seen Michael Jackson, Meat Loaf, Dan Fogelberg, Alice Cooper, and Lynyrd Skynyrd, to name a few. Once isn't enough, either. I've seen Journey several times and more Prince shows than I can count. In the past the thunderous noise never bothered me. I fact, I enjoyed the residual head-buzz from the deafening shows as well as the faint ringing in my ears the day after a great performance that brought me to my feet.

Joel and John are two of my favorites, and tonight they are playing together. "It's a two-fer," Kevin jokes with me.

Kevin plays Ares, my half-brother and nemesis on the show. He and Geoff are both guys' guys—easygoing and relaxed. We get to our seats, right up front, and Kevin and Geoff are audibly impressed, patting me on the back in appreciation. Sam is just as excited as we are. Billy Joel was her first album and her first concert at Madison Square Garden. (Since then she had seen only three concerts!)

The show is amazing, with dueling pianos and two consummate showmen, each with his own style. It is a feast for the eyes and ears. The music, songs we all know and love, is awesome.

But I'd expected too much from myself. Midway through the concert the sound becomes piercing. The searing pain inside my skull moves in so quickly that I don't know what hit me. Suddenly I cannot focus on anything. My dizziness is out of control; the throbbing above my eyes drowns out the music. I grab Sam's arm firmly, and she examines my face for a moment before picking up her jacket to go. I lean over to Kevin. I can barely get out the message that we are leaving, and he is so enthralled with the concert that he can't see the agony I'm in. He simply says he and Geoff can catch a ride home.

With all my effort, I will my legs to carry me. As we get to the exit, passing beyond the direct range of the speakers, the music fades, thankfully. We walk to the other side of the gates and I put my hand on a wall and bend over. *Fuck.* I am just trying to remain upright, hoping nobody can see me. My head is exploding, my mouth is dry and sticky, and my body cold and clammy. I'm going to puke.

Sam is right beside me, with her hand stroking my back. "Tell me what's wrong."

"I don't know. I think I'm having another stroke. I'm so light-headed, Sam. My pulse is racing. I'm going to vomit. I can't seem to catch my breath." I dry heave into my throat and abstractedly notice that I'm trembling.

"Okay, calm down. Take a deep breath in," she says.

I suck in as much air as I can and then let it out, like a prayer. I glance around and notice—no one watching me. Of course not. They are all normal people: inside, enjoying a fabulous concert. It's only Sam and me out here with my demons.

"You're breathing fine. Can you still see?"

I feel the concern in her voice. "Yes, but my head . . . this feels like I did when I was in the car, like the first time. The whole world is spinning. And I feel like I'm in an aquarium. *Again*, Sam. Same thing again."

Intense fear of another crisis grips me. *What was I thinking?* I had arranged for the concert tickets with an unrealistic, consuming desire to resume my life. I wasn't considering any consequences. It's a Friday night, and I was supposed to be taking Sam on a date. *Some date.*

"Kevin, lean on me and we'll walk to the car. You are not having another stroke. There is no cause for one out of the blue like this. Trust me."

"My head is burning. You have no idea."

"It's the noise and the lights. It was just too much. We'll get you home so you can rest. Unless you want to go to the hospital?"

I don't answer. Sam suggesting the hospital is a gauntlet. At times like this I resent her know-it-all attitude. "Hospital?" is *always* the looming question. Back in September last year, when I had my initial symptoms, I saw *several* different doctors who reassured me in *several* different ways, and I didn't go to the hospital until it was *too late*. Would I be too late again this time, or is this time something truly banal? She can't possibly *know*, but can she know *better than I do*? I hate her confidence, and I simultaneously despise myself for questioning her.

Cowed by my fear of hospitals, I put my arm around Sam's shoulders and we walk slowly to the car. The earth comes up to meet my feet with each step, making me stumble.

During the car ride home I calm a bit, wrestling my symptoms into manageable entities. Together, they are truly overwhelming, but once I identify them separately, they are simply the familiar foes, intensified by the concert. Sam, drat her, is probably right—again.

I get into bed and struggle to sleep despite the flashes behind my eyes. Over the past half-year these have largely abated as my brain slowly grappled and regained itself, absorbing its injuries. When it is really taxed, though, all the old symptoms come rushing in again. Tonight is one of those nights.

In fact, the entire weekend is one of those times. I spend the next two days on the couch in our insulated, quiet, windowless room, in front of the TV, waiting to receive my pardon, my stay of execution. Then, before I know it, I am simply praying that I will be well enough for work on Monday.

I cannot miss work. Clearly, work is all I have. I don't have sports. I don't have reading. I don't have concerts. I don't have much of a life except the few hours a day when I pretend to be someone healthy and strong. Monday arrives, my symptoms have eased their vice-grip, and I go through the motions as my phony alter ego.

I am realistic about this: I need the show. If I can't do the show, I might as well kiss my entire career goodbye. One cannot recover from that kind of thing. The unforgiving industry equates dropping out of a show to a betrayal, and I equate my career with my life. The fact that we're both wrong is irrelevant.

THE ALTERNATIVES

Right before I got sick I was part of a unique event that changed me. The big publicity tour for *Kull* that took me through eight cities in seven jam-packed days ended in Minneapolis. Officials in my hometown of Mound, Minnesota, had planned a welcoming event, complete with a park dedication in my name and also the renaming of Forest Lane, the street I grew up on, to Sorbo Lane. (The sign has been stolen so many times that they've stopped replacing it!) As a special part of the ceremony, the Raptor Center at the University of Minnesota asked if I would consider being part of a ceremony to release a bald eagle back into the wild. It had been found with a broken wing, but throughout its rehabilitation the handlers and vets had not domesticated it. This eagle release was momentous proof that mankind can help the species without interfering with it. Many news vans joined a crowd of thousands to witness the event.

I put on heavy leather gloves. Raptor Center representatives taught me to hold the large bird on its back, with my right arm wrapped under and around her wings and my left hand holding her tethered claws. The eagle also wore a snug leather mask over her head. Temporarily removing her eyesight calmed her.

They placed the precious raptor in my waiting arms. The sheer power in this magnificent creature blew my mind. The handler unfettered her feet, removed the mask, and stepped back quickly. I felt the shift of the bird's intensity. Her wings became enormous coils, tense and waiting to be sprung; her claws fiercely gripped my gloved hand. With a countdown from the crowd, my right arm thrust upward as I released her feet with my left hand, launching her into the air.

We all watched in humble awe at her amazing power as she quickly unfurled her eight-foot wingspan and took flight. Whoosh, she stroked downward propelling herself through the air. Whoosh, she covered another fifteen feet, gaining altitude as well. Whoosh, off into the distance.

Hundreds of children ran with pure joy, looking up at this beautiful eagle as she rose into the sky. They shouted and laughed. I smiled, shedding a tear as she disappeared into the distance, above and beyond the trees.

Like most of the crowd, I was filled with reverence for the graceful strength of this creature and for the freedom her flight represented. I had no inkling that my own captivity was fast approaching. In the weeks, months, and years after my crisis I would often think back to that moment and wish for some of that bird's impressive power. I dreamt of getting my wings back someday.

In Auckland, away from my US medical experts, Sam and I searched under every rock for alternative healers. (My doctors' timelines were exhausted and I defied their prognostications—they had no more advice for me.)

Because many of my issues originated from my compromised eyesight, we met with an eye guy named Gunter. His office was located in a chic, hip suburb of Auckland called Ponsonby.

Gunter was German, slightly built with thinning hair and an intense demeanor. He was intrigued as I related the events that led me there, but by now I was tired of astonishing people with my story; I preferred for them to shock me with a cure. Gunter told me he used to wear coke bottle–thick glasses until he discovered the Bates Method, which he would share with me. He said he could teach me to see fully, even with my brain compromised by stroke.

Sight consists of a pathway, Gunter explained, defined primarily by the optic nerve, which runs from the back of the eye into the brain. Muscles acting upon the nerve can decrease its efficacy. Most people see with the front of their eyes, meaning they see on the surface of things, but he wanted to teach me how to see with my mind, from the back of my brain via the optic nerve. If we could free up the nerve, we could improve my vision. We did relaxation exercises for about an hour to teach me to identify my optic nerve and use it.

Then he showed me a computer-generated image. He asked me to look through it, to see it with the back of my mind. If I could unfocus my eyes on the image, it would become three-dimensional. This was an exercise in control—or rather lack of control. If I could stop trying so hard and let my vision do its thing, it would naturally improve. He gave me some large 3-D pictures to practice with and asked me to come back in a week.

Sam and I got in the car to drive home. "What did you think?" she asked.

"I don't know. It seems like bullshit, but maybe there is something to it. I can't really do that 3-D thing. Can you?"

"It's really hard until you know the trick. Then it's much easier. I'm not sure how that could translate to real life, though. But I guess the exercise is useful somehow."

"Yeah . . . I wish I knew how, though. Wow, I'm tired, Sam. I hope that's a good sign."

My follow-up visit proved unenlightening, but I wanted to give it time to work, so I kept going back every week for a few months. If anything, I found the sessions relaxing and the exercises took my mind off of my mind. The whole looking *through* pictures and popping out the 3-D images hidden there started to actually work, which was a minor triumph, but in the end I wasn't completely sold on the idea that this would really improve my vision. I mean, my vision loss was a big black hole. I had been hopeful that the exercises might eventually train my brain to fill in the hole rather than be so confused by it.

I got burned out on seeing doctors all the time. If they didn't offer drastic change or improvement (and they never did), I dropped them.

Patricia, Eric's wife, called me when she heard that I was suffering from migraines. "I have a doctor who is phenomenal. He's a cranial-sacral therapist. He's so good, he doesn't take any new patients, but I have a standing appointment with him on Wednesday if you want it."

"What does he do?"

"He manipulates your scalp and your tail bone, very, very gently. He's not a chiropractor. You really should see him, Kevin. Trust me."

Patricia is a very bright lady, so I took her advice seriously. I went to see the guy that Wednesday after work.

Dr. Tony Norie's office, on the ground floor of an apartment building, had a full waiting room. I could feel the atmosphere change when I entered the room: As a local Auckland "celebrity," I was used to causing a stir. However, I hoped these patients were there for the other names on the door; my patience was frayed. For this new, unfamiliar doctor, I did not want to hang out in a crowded waiting room, enduring surreptitious glances and outright stares. I had become increasingly self-conscious about my handicap, particularly in medical settings. I felt like people saw right into my vulnerability.

After the patient in front of me finished at the reception desk, I checked in. Lucky for me, I was immediately shown into a small white room where there was a plain treatment bed with white sheets on it.

Dr. Norie introduced himself as he walked briskly into the examination room. He stood about five-foot-ten, but his powerful presence made him seem taller. He sat on a rolling stool and I told him my story.

He took a moment to gather his thoughts. "I can help you," he said. "I know I can, but only if you want to be helped."

"Of course I want help. Why else would I be here?"

"Kevin, sometimes after people get hurt, that pain gets entirely enmeshed with who they are, and they get comfortable in their new identity of a sufferer seeking relief. It's a vicious cycle. This thing you have is powerful, and it would be easy to become 'the guy looking for help' instead of 'the guy who heals himself.'"

"Okay, I am the guy who is healing himself," I answered, mildly perturbed. I didn't much like the guy challenging me like that, but I was desperate for him to be what he thought he could be. It had been a long day, and my symptoms, never much fun, were particularly present in this bright, antiseptic environment.

"I can turn the lights off if you'd like. The sun is still bright enough for our purposes."

How did he know? It didn't matter. That small gesture rekindled my hope that I could trust him. "Sure. That'd be great. Thanks."

"Let's get started. Please remove your shoes and lie on your back."

I lay down and he positioned himself at my head, which he gently but firmly lifted and held.

His hands were spread out over my skull, moving only minutely. "Can you tell me what this dent is from?" he asked, referring to the large flat area on the back of my head.

"Shortly after I was born, my mom caught my sister, Pam, throwing potatoes at me in the crib. She may have dropped me on my head. I was the new baby in the house and I was told my sister didn't like losing the title 'baby of the house.' That's the only story I have, and I'm not sure about it."

"Okay. So, you've had it all your life."

"Pretty much." I felt a tingling down my leg. I had been getting sciatica recently, but I hadn't mentioned that to him.

"You should be feeling some tingling down your left leg."

"Yeah . . ." Wow, this was something else. He was only touching my head, and it kind of freaked me out.

"After I'm done tonight, you're going to pee like a racehorse. When you get home, you'll need the toilet for a while, and then you will feel much better. I'm releasing the toxins through your bowels. Just relax now."

That was easy to do. The lights were low, I was tired, and the gentle pressure on my head put me in a meditative state. After a few minutes he spoke again in a soft voice.

"Kevin, if you were given a gift, would you stomp on it and throw it away?"

"What? Of course not," I answered, confused.

Then he quietly told me, "This illness is a gift you have been given. It is not to be discarded like moldy bread. Use it and let it help you."

After I returned home (and used the toilet for all it was worth) I told this story to Sam. She burst into tears. She was amazed and grateful that someone would risk laying out the truth in that way. Sam said she had tried to get that message across to me but finally realized I simply couldn't hear it from her.

Even moldy bread can give you penicillin, but you have to have the recipe. Dr. Norie charged me with making that recipe for myself.

FEAR

REFLECTING ON DR. NORIE'S ADVICE reminded me of Dr. Stutz—and my elusive shadow.

It is only eight weeks into my convalescence. During our second meeting I sit in the chair opposite Dr. Stutz. He reiterates his assessment from our previous visit, and then asks me how I am doing with his advice.

I don't quite know how to frame it but . . . I can't get my head around the concept of the shadow, much less embrace it. (Frankly, at this point I am still trying to come to grips with having to sit down to use the toilet efficiently.)

I turn to my yellow legal pad and the list scribbled there: notes from the several times I listened to the tape of our first appointment. "Number one: my body wants to work out, but I just don't have the energy. Then I get this heavy, shaking, nauseous feeling from *not* going to work out. So I go to bed, but my brain just races. It won't quit. Then, when I finally do fall asleep, I sleep, like, fourteen hours."

Stutz, calm and intense, leans forward with his elbows on his knees. He thinks for a moment before beginning. "John Wooden—you know who he is, right?"

I nod *of course*. One of the winningest college basketball coaches ever, he is a hero of mine.

"Well, before he started winning, he used to lose. His team would be unbeatable during the season, but then he drove them too hard at the end and they'd be defeated. He realized he was fucking up his own team.

"After he figured that out he laid back. *No* practice during the final four! And they started winning.

"Some sprinters—there are sprinters who are good: explosive, strong—and then there are the great ones. Those are the guys who can relax. It's almost like they give up in the middle of the race. By doing less, by just relying on the past work, they get more strength."

He pauses to look at me. I must have a blank expression on my face because he continues, "It's counterintuitive, but only because you are dealing on a purely *physical* level. At some point you'll realize it's more than that . . ."

I shift in my chair. I want to hear—really *hear and understand* what he is saying—but my symptoms hound me.

Stutz presses on: "I'm working with one actor now, actually, who's on set with an older, established director. This director, he won't let the actor do his whole prep thing to get into character and stuff. He distracts him from it until he says, 'action.' It drives the guy crazy, but at the end of the shoot, seeing his dailies, he tells me his performance is good—better, even. It's because he's done the work, and the director understands it's time to relax, so he forces the actor to lay off." He pauses to see if it is sinking in.

I hope I look convinced, because I'm not. I look down at my sad catalog of scribbles.

"I guess I just want that comfort zone to know that I'm going to be 100 percent again. I have this great fear of relapsing. Like, you know they put this coil inside," I place my hand on my shoulder, over the disappeared lump, "and I don't like it there. I just, you know, want the fucking thing out."

Stutz nods, then shrugs. "I hope it stays there, to remind you not to be a *schmuck*."

Wow. Okay. I never thought of it like *that*.

"My doctor says for me to jog, like, work it off. But my body says no way, stop."

"Who is that again?"

"Huizenga. He was the doctor for the . . ."

"Right, for the Raiders, the team doctor. Doctors are . . . they know one side of it. I'm telling you that you're fucking yourself if you try to push through."

"By doing less, I'm getting stronger." I speak it like the moral of an unlikely fable—but I don't buy it for a second.

"You have to take a long view of time. Physically, your body will come back when you start working out again. You'll see, because the groundwork is there. But your way of thinking about it is fucked up. You push yourself too hard."

Stutz takes a breath in, nodding. "The fear of relapse is just a metaphor for loss of control. But your loss is not a bad thing—it's a good thing. You've released a bit of your desire to control your physical world—your body—but you still crave control of the spirit world, the emotional stuff. Look, some people don't believe in God, but you do and that's good. You need to turn to God in a constructive manner. Create a relationship with God every day. Pray every day. Did we talk about the Grateful Flow?"

"Um . . ." I am not sure if I remember that or not.

Stutz becomes slightly more conversational, leaning back toward me, but there is nothing careless about him. "So, the Grateful Flow is like a prayer. You give thanks for things—it can be anything, really. Little things, like, I like hot water, so I'm thankful for my hot shower in the morning. I'm grateful the car started. Don't repeat stuff, though, because then it just becomes a litany, and that's not what this is about. So you say the things you are grateful for, and you'll start to feel it in your body, like your third eye. Then you'll want to create another thought, but don't let yourself. Stop the exercise there and then wait. That pure energy is what you are looking for—not thought. The goal is the energy of the flow. Then pray, just for wisdom and a silent mind." He waits a bit before continuing. "This is a master tool to control the mind."

I immediately focus on the contradiction: Control the mind, but do not be in control. His face is serious.

"You put your mind at one with the flow of a positive and moving universe."

Okay, now that makes more sense.

Then he says the clincher: "You cannot solve a disease of thought—a spinning mind—with more thoughts. It won't work."

I nod. "Yeah. Like I see that I overprepare. I have to know all the lines in the scene, and I have to pore over the scripts and think of every contingency. I know it's too much . . ."

Stutz smiles and nods warmly, although he is all business. I do not really get everything he says, but I know, intrinsically, that he is hitting the nail on the head. "It takes balls to do *less*. You can't intellectualize this. Do less—and the shadow will do more. Close your eyes for a minute."

With my eyes shut, Stutz guides me through a short visualization, something I have done countless times in acting class. He instructs me to remember a time, maybe when I was a child, when I felt weak and out of control.

I am about ten or eleven, and my brothers are picking teams for a game of basketball. Al is five years older than me and Tom is a year younger than him. They pick my neighbor and good friend, Mark. We are comparable athletes. I cannot understand why they choose Mark over me. I am disappointed, hurt, and jealous.

Stutz speaks softly into my reverie. "That's your shadow—a source of insecurity and jealousy. How do you suppose it influenced you?"

Um . . . I knew that I was capable. I always wanted to lead, but I never quite performed well enough. Like in high school—I could have been the quarterback, but I was content to be the runner. I played both sides, offence and defense, but only just adequately. I didn't want to shine too brightly. I am disgusted with myself for holding myself back from performing better athletically.

"Why did the shadow hold you back?"

Fear.

Fear of success.

Fear of failure, of making a fool of myself.

"That's right. Inside, you preferred to fly under the radar. You didn't want people to see the insecure, jealous, shadow part. Now your carefully constructed façade is fractured and the shadow wants to be brought into the spotlight.

"You need to talk to him every day and invite him into your life. Bring your fear into the open. Look at it. Examine it even, and you will see it is not 'real'—it is not tangible. Okay, you can open your eyes again.

"Like the boxer who, even if he wins, goes back to the locker room and hits himself in the head for all the mistakes he made during the fight? When something bad happens, don't beat yourself up. Beating yourself up is a sin; it's overindulgent. The grateful flow is a tool to control that. It helps to calm the mind and free it. I do it often, like when I'm standing in line at the bank. Otherwise, I'd just be thinking idle thoughts. It is an inevitable human conceit that our thoughts are important. Mostly, however, they are not."

The tape clicks off, ending our hour. Stutz looks at me with penetrating eyes, waiting for me to acknowledge his final insight, I suppose. I nod my appreciation and look down a final time at my list. I have checked off all my notes, save one. "I just hope I go back to feeling good again."

"You have to work hard to get peace of mind."

RAGE

EVEN THOUGH I KNEW Stutz had a point—and I was trying to let go—I just couldn't shake the suspicion that my progress was too slow. Head injuries manifest in countless different ways, but the most common symptom for a head-injured patient is an enhanced or uncontrollable temper, an accelerated rage response. I had that one, for sure. Basically, my emotions were not my own. I have always been impatient, but now, with my temper constantly burning at medium-high, I was rude and overly critical much of the time.

I just wanted health. I became irritated and unreasonable, even with Sam, who was constantly offering me more help than I ever dreamed I would need from anyone—more help than I ever *wanted* to need. She was always optimistic (read: *annoying*) and usually had logical explanations for my latest symptoms (read: *ridiculous rationalizations I was unprepared to accept*). I typically rejected her viewpoint, though I admit now those were not my finest moments.

Lucky for me, Sam isn't superficial, but she's also not a carpet. Sam basically put up with this new me. She understood that the anger and the nastiness that oozed out of me was the head injury talking. She knew I was in pain most of the time. Thankfully, her patience was a lot better than mine had ever been.

I received an invitation to host the Miss World pageant in London. I wanted to do it. I love London. It promised to be an exciting trip—and a fantastic opportunity for exposure on a world-renowned television extravaganza. Plus, I was married, not dead.

Sam and I discussed it over dinner. She gently but steadfastly discouraged me. The flight alone would trash me, she warned. I joked that she just didn't want me socializing with all those beautiful babes, but I admitted to myself that my condition was tenuous at best. Sam always enjoyed talking things out, evaluating, but I did not care to hear her reiterate how incapable I was at dealing with the most mundane things, like airplanes and jetlag. My illness was running the show and that angered me.

"Fine, enough. I get it! Just drop it, already."

My words sounded harsh, even to me. Sam ceased her commentary. She cleared the dishes and went into the kitchen.

I grabbed my jacket, realizing the time. "Hey, c'mon. We better go or we'll be late."

We had tickets to a friend's play, and as usual, I was dreading having an episode while we were out. My symptoms were an erratic tide: Sometimes they would thankfully ebb, but other times they would surge, rendering me completely vulnerable. I imagined this scenario during intermission, when we were certain to see friends and acquaintances. (I could never go out without running into people I knew or who knew me.) Being private about my condition gave me little leeway in the public arena. If I wasn't doing well, I would smile and nod along with the conversation, all the while hoping I didn't just hurl on the person I was talking to and waiting for an opportune moment to disengage myself and leave. At those times I would nudge Sam, silently willing her to take the hint and justify our departure. I couldn't do it myself. I couldn't come up with an excuse that sounded plausible to me. It was crucial for me that no one knew how weak I really was, and so, particularly in those moments, I just became a good actor who was miserable at improvisation.

I was already waiting in the passenger seat as Sam got in the car. "It's about time. What were you doing in there?" I said in as friendly a way as I could muster (i.e., not very).

"I just had to clean up in the kitchen, put away the leftovers. Then I realized I forgot to put on mascara."

"Well, we're late now. Why didn't you put it on when you were getting dressed?" I could not conceal my impatience and anxiety.

"I just told you. I forgot. Never mind. It's done now. And we'll be right on time." She put the keys in the ignition.

"We'll be late!" I argued. "It'll take at least ten minutes to get there, and then we won't find a parking spot."

"There's a *positive* thought! We've got twenty minutes before show time, if they even start on time. Plus, you have no idea how good I am at conjuring up parking spaces."

"I just hate to be late. You know that," I grumbled. It was true. If there was any weak link in our relationship, aside from my condition, it was that I was always five minutes early, and she was inevitably five minutes late. I had chided her on this point more than once. This time was the straw that broke the camel's back.

She jolted the car back in park, halfway down the drive. "Yes, I know that. Why don't you just go ahead then? I don't need to go. I'll be inside."

Seething, she calmly got out of the car as I answered, "I'm already too late!" Oh, she was aggravating! She didn't even look back before she walked into the house, closing the door behind her.

I shut off the car and followed her inside. She was sitting on the stairs in the entry, her head in her hands. "Sam, quit acting like a child and let's go."

"Me acting like a child? Me?! Look at yourself! 'Waa! I can't go jogging anymore! Waa! I wish I could have hosted *Saturday Night Live* when they called. Waa! Waa! I can't go to London for a beauty contest!' You're constantly complaining! You're never happy and I can't take it anymore!"

I snatched the bait. "I'm not complaining! I'm stating the facts! That's all true and more! It's so aggravating, being like this—unable to do stuff! You should try it sometime, and you'd understand!"

"Well, I can't. 'Waa! Nobody understands me!'"

"You know what? Maybe this isn't working. Maybe you should just leave." I slammed the front door shut for emphasis. "I mean, what's the point? We don't even get along. You get me so angry! Maybe it's time to call the lawyers." I went over to the living room and sat down.

"Yes, that's perfect. It's the end of our marriage now because I had the audacity to voice an opinion—no—because I was late getting ready for a stupid play you don't even want to go to!"

"Well, you're obviously not happy, so why are you still here? You're miserable, I'm miserable. Maybe we just aren't meant to be together."

She walked to the doorway of the living room and folded her arms, laughing through her tears. "Kevin, I understand that you're in pain and that you're scared. But honestly? Really? You're done?"

"I don't know, Sam. If you're so unhappy . . ."

"I'm unhappy because you are. Most of the time, when you're not around, I'm pretty good."

I stood up, feeling vindicated. "So *I'm* the downer? This is all *my fault!* Perfect! You're unhappy being with me."

"Can you blame me? Look at you! Nothing is ever right anymore! Can't you just appreciate that you're alive at least? Can't you just be thankful that you still have your left arm and can play *some* golf, even if it's not the best golf of your life? You could have lost your leg, you could have ended up a complete vegetable, Kevin, but you didn't! You're here, you're still working. But all you can do is worry and whine about stupid beauty contests—things you don't have." She was crying. I glared at her, enraged by the barrage of emotion coming at me.

"It's not just this beauty contest! It's everything! It's taking over my life, Sam. You don't understand—you're healthy!"

"It's a *part* of your life, not the whole thing, Kevin! You have so much! You're going to let a beauty contest ruin your evening?"

"I was ready to go. I was fine!"

"You were *miserable* all through dinner! You think that was fun for me? Listening to you complaining the whole evening? Was it fun for you?" She shook her head. "I can't do *that* anymore. I can't be your cheerleader if you keep throwing rotten eggs at me."

"You're right. I'm miserable, but I have a right to be!"

"Sure! You have every right. Just don't take it out on me!"

I answered the only thing that came to my mind. "Fine! I'm sorry!"

"Well, sorry isn't going to cut it." She pointed at me, accusingly. "You need to learn how to be happy or else you're going to kill any hope either of us have to lead a normal life again." Her hands went to her hips. Her face was red and shiny, the mascara making fugitive streaks down her beautiful cheeks. "And I want that. I don't need fantastic, but normal would be good. Average, okay. I want it for you. I want you to be the happy guy I met two years ago." She drew a staggered breath in and then sobbed, "I want to be happy *for* you!" She left the room in silence.

There would be no play that night; there was enough drama at home.

I sat down again in the living room to contemplate what had just happened: our first *real* fight as a married couple. The subject matter couldn't be more raw. I took some time to figure out how to react to what she had said.

Did she even have a point, or was she just going off half-cocked? I was miserable, truly, but wasn't I justified? I was depressed and hopeless. Why shouldn't I be? I had had the world at my feet. *Hercules* was a worldwide hit. I finally had a movie career growing. And now it was stripped away from me. I was living a lie, pretending to be normal when I could barely get through six hours a day on set. I laid my head back on the top of the couch and thought about all the reasons I had to be sad.

Then I started thinking about what happy might be like, and I realized that she was dead-on. Miserable wasn't any way to live life. I needed an attitude makeover, but I had no idea how to get one.

Maybe she knew.

I found her, clean-faced with PJs on, in our TV room reading her book. I sat down on the couch, nudging her over to make room for me. I knew she liked that. She often told me she liked my size because I made her feel petite, and at five-foot-ten, there weren't a lot of guys who could do that. I knew I had to ingratiate myself for my apology, and this small gesture worked. Sam smiled at me, albeit with some residual tears in her eyes.

"I'm sorry," I began. Then, I couldn't continue. I felt like such a failure, and I couldn't even confide that to Sam—she might interpret it as her own.

"I know. Me too. I flew off the handle. I'm not sure why that happened."

"You're doing too much, Sam," I offered.

"No, listen: You need to lighten up. Your impatience is eating at you, and that's hurting your recovery, not to mention our relationship. Trust me. You will get better—slowly. We've seen improvement—month to month, not day by day. Do you see the improvement from that first day to where you are now? You are getting better, and you have to trust that."

"It's hard," I shrugged.

"Of course it is. Anything worth fighting for is never easy." She reached out to me and I turned and enveloped her in a strong, meaningful hug.

"Remember the grateful prayer Stutz gave you?" she asked, with her head cradled on my shoulder.

"Yeah."

"Well, work it, baby, 'cause you've got a lot to be thankful for. Every day, when you wake up, just be thankful for *that*, for the hot shower, for the small reprieves, for the rays of hope."

As if on cue, Gizmoe sneezed. "For Gizmoe," I said.

Sam's smile whispered on my neck. "I know it's hard, but you have the strength to do this. You are the strongest man I know."

"I know. I'm Hercules," I scoffed quietly. I had lost so much of my muscle mass, and although I had regained some since the hospital, I didn't have the drive or the stamina to recreate the heft, the brute physicality I used to have.

Sam must have sensed my thoughts. She pushed me back so she could look in my eyes, and she took my face in her gentle hands.

"Stop that," she scolded. "More so now than ever, Kevin, you are the strongest man I know. And I love you madly."

"I love you too. I'll work on this. I'm going to beat this thing," I promised, still uncertain if I could deliver.

"Embrace it instead, Kevin."

No, not that again. I didn't know how, couldn't understand why, and certainly did not want to. This illness was my mortal enemy. How would I ever embrace that?

I frowned and tried to shrug it away. "Now remember what Dr. Wong advised me?" I scolded, "Nah too much ee-moh-shun!" I did a very poor Chinese accent. "See? You ah bad fo' me, get me aw emotional!"

She laughed. "You're right. I'm sorry."

"You should be." I kissed her cheek, tasting the salty wetness there. "But I'm gonna let you make it up to me. Come on. We might as well blow all the circuits while we're at it."

Laughing, she clumsily marked her book with one hand because I held her other wrist (I wasn't about to let go) as she followed me into the dark bedroom.

PART III
WHOLLY HUMAN

FREEDOM

AUCKLAND WEATHER IS ISLAND WEATHER. They say "dress for three seasons" because it is so changeable. "If you don't like the weather, wait five minutes."

One weekend, as a little getaway, Sam and I went to a romantic hotel that consisted of a collection of bungalows nestled on a forest hillside.

The hotel restaurant had large, plate-glass windows on two sides, giving us diners a dreamy view of the scattered cabins with their corrugated metal roofs. Halfway through dinner it began to rain, with rolling thunder in the distance. Soon, the rain turned into a deluge. Copious raindrops and low-lying clouds obscured our view. The thunder roared, all the other buildings disappeared, and abruptly we became the last people on earth.

Suddenly a lightning bolt struck very, very close by, charging the air. The entire restaurant fell silent. We all glanced around, expecting to see fire somewhere. I looked at Sam. "Wow. That was really close! Giz probably won't have liked that."

She looked at me, concerned. "Oh my gosh, I bet she's totally freaked out."

We quickly finished eating and headed back to our cabin, heedless of the rain. I opened the door, and a trembling Giz skulked out from under the bed to greet us. She didn't sleep at all that night, and after that she was always a basket case in thunderstorms.

For the rest of her life I became her go-to guy for every rainstorm. She would seek me out, tremulous, demanding my comfort and security. Gizmoe recognized a strength in me. She couldn't know the rain was just water, condensation in an endless cycle, but she trusted that I could protect her and keep her safe.

I've heard that He won't lead you to it if He can't get you through it, and I guess I started thinking that sounded reasonable, if the Gizmoe analogy was any guide. If I was just a puppy, afraid of the rain, maybe my God was looking out for me after all.

My hurricane had hit a full half-year before, and it was still raining pretty hard in my life. I struggled every day, working very limited hours. But compared to what I had already experienced, Sam was right: I had come a long way, and my symptoms were simply the tempest, a part of me I ought to accept.

I needed help to do that. I rededicated myself to finding a way to God through prayer. I decided to start praying simply for faith, for humility, and for a vision of things working out alright. I longed to hear His gentle voice again, like a child yearns for his daddy's reassurance on a dark night, like Giz seeking out my warm comfort.

First, I asked Him for an umbrella.

After the knock-down, drag-out fight with Sam, I realized I needed to drop my bad attitude. My illness was what it was, and thinking negatively was only hurting me further. Dr. Norie and Dr. Stutz had both advised me to embrace my illness, but I rejected their advice because I couldn't understand why or how. Now Sam was urging the same notion, but there was even more at stake: my marriage. I determined to take a more positive approach.

True, my attitude was ridiculously impracticable. But it was an iceberg of habit—I needed a quick thaw, maybe a nuke . . . or at least a global warming trend.

I started with a new mantra, five times out loud each morning: "I'm getting better and better every day." Although this was difficult to believe on the days I suffered relapses, on better days the tune obligated me to appreciate my improvement.

I was stronger and feeling better for longer periods. Even my ability to handle strong feelings had improved. Although most of the time sex felt like it would kill me, it was finally sinking in that I wasn't dead yet.

The depression was steadily lifting as my brain healed, lightening my outlook. Sam's resonant optimism broke through, past the doctors' voices and their warnings that there might be no more improvement after three months. Recognizing that I had already proved the doctors wrong augmented my confidence.

My perspective shifted. I saw myself on an uphill trend and with a way out, one that the doctors' prognoses had obscured. It finally crystallized: Their word was not gospel. Sure, they had saved my life, but that was then.

Most of my friends did not comprehend all the details of my troubles. This was partly because of the secrecy issue but also because sharing this frail side of myself with others had been too difficult. Even my parents were so far away, both physically and in understanding. I was in this alone with Sam and with God, but God helps those who help themselves. So getting better was just up to me. I gradually began to try to lead instead of follow, beg, and succumb.

I wasn't going to give the bastards anything, and I was going to take back what they had stolen from me. I was angry at the strokes, but I finally figured out that they had no *real* power.

It wasn't so much about *healing* as being *happy*.

I began using my grateful prayer again.

I thanked Him for the voice that September day. Although I didn't heed the warning, I wondered if He could have done it simply to let me know He was there. Perhaps that was blessing enough.

I thanked Him for the small reprieves: the gratifying workouts and good sleeps at night. I thanked Him for saving my arm, my speech, and what I had left of my sight. I thanked Him for Sam and Giz, who had come into my life at just the right moment. And for the character of Hercules, who was saving my life. I had defined myself by my job, so I thanked Him that I still had one. And although I would never measure up to Hercules's physical strength, I borrowed his stamina for my everyday battle just to live a normal life.

My illness made me special—in a way that I never wanted nor expected, yes, but if I was to be special, then I was going to do something with that gift. I wasn't a half-god or any part god. I was a mere mortal, with human limitations and problems, but I was determined not to behave like a victim anymore.

NEW FRONTIER

BY THE SPRING OF 1999, over a year and a half after I first fell ill, I was back up to working some eight-hour days, and I could fake feeling well for at least that long. The humming was still there, but it had calmed and I had also grown accustomed to it. I could drive again, although I almost never did. In short, I had learned to manage my issues. My prospects were looking up, even as lingering symptoms often tried to convince me otherwise.

One day Majel Roddenberry, *Star Trek* creator Gene Roddenberry's widow, called to tell me about a few other sci-fi scripts her late husband had written. I couldn't believe that I was talking to Majel Roddenberry, Nurse Chapel from *Star Trek*—the woman with the turbo-bra! Madonna had nothing on her. I admit it, I'm more than a bit of a Trekkie, if having seen every episode a minimum of twenty times qualifies me. No, I don't dress up and go to Trek conventions, but short of that . . . I loved that show. My brothers and I would get into heated arguments about the significance of certain events, like whether time would revert back to exactly how it had been if a single event was simply postponed for a few months by some time-traveling meddlers. (See what I mean?) We all relished the particular cheesiness of that groundbreaking show.

Suffice it to say, Majel had my attention. She wanted us to develop one of Gene's works into a new series. I immediately told her to send me the scripts and I would look them over. "Now we'll need to do a better job on the special effects," I ventured. She laughed, and we ended the conversation promising to meet on my next trip to LA.

After I read the scripts I called Majel and suggested we could take the standout ideas from the two best scripts and merge them into one show. She loved the idea, and next thing I knew, I got a call from Dick Askin, president of programming for Tribune Television, saying he was sending one of his top producers down to New Zealand to talk about the new series.

Karen Corbin was a petite brunette with a calm, serious demeanor. We met her for dinner at my favorite restaurant, the Olympic Café. (I did not choose it for its name, by the way; it just happened to be one of the best restaurants in Auckland. It also didn't hurt that they made the greatest bread pudding known to mankind.)

Karen had flown a long way to seal the deal, but the dinner was a formality; they wanted me and I wanted them. We conversed comfortably about how the show would be conceived. Called *Gene Roddenberry's Andromeda*, it would be another space frontier show like *Star Trek*, but it would be even farther into the future. I'd play Dylan Hunt, the captain of a ship who is lost in a time warp far into my own future. He's lost his life as he knew it and has to find his way in this new era, like a fish out of water. Something about his story appealed to me on a very emotional level. We discussed the journey of my character and the intent of the show—its message. I wanted to be sure it was a family show: wholesome, expressing good values and positive ideas. Karen agreed and seemed genuinely devoted to producing the best show possible.

We made a tacit agreement to let the lawyers duke it out over the particulars.

In the meantime Rob Tapert and Eric Gruendemann came to my camper to discuss continuing with *Hercules* for another three years.

It was warm and cramped in my camper, and as usual, I was having a challenging day. Rob, clearly uncomfortable in the close quarters, sat opposite me at the yellow Formica table. Eric, beside him, seemed to be along as chaperone.

Rob had done the research and found that although Universal might not be interested in keeping the show alive after seven years, there were syndicated outlets that would finance a few more years of episodes. He pitched his case: "The show is still viable, sir. Universal is being ridiculous, but their new regime just won't support any old product, even our number-one show. As much money as we're already going to see on the back end, we can make even more from doing three more years and owning them outright. Now that we've organized production around your limited schedule, your workload can continue to be exactly what you've wanted. Your illness, or whatever, won't be a hazard for us."

As he spoke I felt the anger rise inside me. I never wanted this: to be grateful that I could stumble through an exhausting ten-hour day. It was as if my health issues were simply stumbling blocks that he had somehow magnificently surmounted. I wished, unkindly, that I could shove my brain into his skull for one day, to have him feel what I was going through. Then he might not treat it so cavalierly.

Rob often waltzed in when he needed me, feigning concern and interest. I remembered the time not long before when he approached me to write a second letter to studio heads in support of the newest spin-off, *Young Hercules*. He was amiable and considerate as he indicated what he wanted me to write. Suddenly he scrutinized my face and asked, "I see they are having you grow stubble for this episode? It looks good."

I eyed him, incredulous. I really didn't want to hand my boss a "sign" (à la Jeff Foxworthy), but my sarcastic side insisted: "Rob, I've had stubble for this character since the very first movie. It's only been four years."

It really is too bad that things had gotten so sour between us. Together with the other powers at the studio, Rob had given me the part of a lifetime, including a TV family and adopted country that yet holds a special place in my heart. But once the first spin-off started, my crew began complaining to me that *Hercules* was being given short shrift for the benefit of the other show—Rob's fiancée's show. Aside from losing our directors, department heads divulged to me that they had to fight a lot harder to get the equipment, FX, stunts, and so forth, and they often lost those fights. They apologized to me that their hands were tied. Of course, I had no power over how the finances or materials on the two shows were managed. I did one stunt that was edited out of our final cut because it was "reserved" for the spin-off. Rob also used *Hercules* as a testing ground. For instance, they built a new creature for my show, and four weeks later the spin-off got ten of them, resulting in that show having greater production value than *Hercules*.

My skin itched from Rob's seemingly hollow concern for me and my show. Had he so easily forgotten all our history? *Hercules* created the spin-offs and then was carelessly relegated to the back burner.

Aside from this, my enthusiasm for *Andromeda* was an act of self-preservation. Hercules was a character I loved—and a guy I kind of hated. I had devoted my whole life to him and he had almost killed me, and that still stung, frankly. I needed desperately to move on.

Our contract called for only seven shows in the final season. I told Rob and Eric I could happily finish out the season, the full complement of twenty-two episodes, but I couldn't do more because I had another show starting up. I really wanted to finish out the full season for the fans, more than anything else.

Unfortunately, my response that I could not do another three seasons infuriated Rob. He pushed away from the table and exited my camper, mumbling something unattractive over his shoulder.

Had we been in another setting, I believe Rob and I could have been great friends. I admired his creativity and drive, which mirrored my own, and his business acumen needs no further description. It isn't easy producing a hit show from nothing, and then doing it again and again, and he deserves all the credit for those impressive accomplishments. That our business relationship cost us our friendship may simply be a small thing, I don't know. I regretted our mutual distrust, but there was nothing to be done about it then. The waters ran too deep.

Eric looked at me after Rob stormed off and shrugged, "I told him not to come in here . . ."

Rob decided not to finish the full year of shows. It was disappointing, but predictable.

His decision determined the end date of the series. All of a sudden I got excited about my future: *A change was gonna come.* I had needed a new opportunity on which to focus, and the Gene Roddenberry show was clearly the perfect blessing. It was a chance to shed the past. More than that, it represented an opportunity to reinvent myself—to myself—and to grow as an actor.

My lawyer, Dave, called me to ask what I wanted in the *Andromeda* contract. I said the first thing that came to mind, "I need a golf course nearby."

He laughed. "I'm thinking we should ask for a limited schedule. I can probably get you twelve-hour day, door to door. How about that?"

I had finally relinquished my need to be the invincible, all-capable, strong man enough to rest a bit on my laurels. Before I got sick I was putting in eighteen hours a day door to door with my drive time and my gym schedule factored in. If Dave could get me a limited schedule, I chose to see that as an affirmation of my worth.

Plus, *Andromeda* would have a larger series-regular cast than *Hercules*, which meant there were plenty of characters besides mine that episodes could be written about. I was done being the only guy the show was about, being in every scene and doing every fight.

"Yeah, Dave, twelve hours, door to door. Absolutely, put that in the contract." But I won't lie: The fact that I truly needed this concession still irked me.

There were a couple of other perks that I got. We negotiated for me to direct an episode or two each year. The way I was feeling, I couldn't see it happening (and it never did), but I was still trying to be optimistic. I also got say over final edit, an executive producer credit, final say on cast and directors, and the choice of which Canadian city to shoot in. (They supplied housing and travel as well.) Vancouver was closest to LA as well as my mom and dad in Vegas (and it's still one of my favorite places in the world).

All in all, I got a tremendous deal, but these points were reasonable considerations for someone coming off a show with such a strong track record. Airing in 176 countries, *Hercules* peaked in the ratings during our third season and held the title of Most Watched TV Show in the World for the rest of its run. I was in a good place—on paper, anyway.

When it came to the financial negotiations for *Andromeda*, my new manager told me that no one would ever see a contract like this again in television. I had a forty-four-show guarantee, something very rare and certainly unheard of for a show that didn't even have a pilot! It meant I would get paid for forty-four episodes even if they failed to produce it. In comparison, the *Seinfeld* pilot was rejected, so a studio executive who believed in the show fought to produce three subsequent *Seinfeld* episodes (using part of a budget he had for something else). (It did okay after that!) These days studios produce three, six, or nine shows; guarantees are a thing of the past; and the money has dried up too. In my case Tribune had all the resources lined up and they were ready to make a TV show with me in the lead. Right or wrong, they were banking on me making the show a success.

A MYTHIC ENDING

AFTER SEVEN YEARS today is the last day of filming for *Hercules: The Legendary Journeys*. My show. In one sense I cannot fathom that this day has arrived, and yet I have been anxiously anticipating it since the day, almost two years ago, when my life disintegrated. As I carefully discard the shell of my character, I naively hope to also, finally, exorcise the illness that is so indwelt. The psychological connection I have to this character and this job is a Gordian Knot.

I pour out of bed and stretch, willing the dizziness to abate and the circulating blood to heal my head. Sam puts on a pot of rolled and steel-cut oats, my favorite, and gets out the maple syrup and raisins.

My assistant drives me to set. It is early still, and the winter sun has yet to show its face to this sleepy island world.

I step up into my camper. There's my Hercules outfit, the one I've worn nearly every day for seven years (there have been several copies). I change clothes, pulling on the boots over the woven leather of my pants, tying the yellow chamois vest over the linen undergarment. I run my hands through my hair, a high school habit that has become more pronounced of late as a release for my wearisome nerves. To warm up in the morning chill, I pull on the big fleece robe that wardrobe always leaves me. Stepping back out into the hushed mist, I do a final, somber stroll to the makeup trailer.

I sit in the same old barber chair and Annie puts on my same old makeup. She is quick—years of practice—and moves on to my hair. I scowl at her and she responds with a sparkling laugh. We have a running joke that she puts too much crap in my hair, but she always manages to goop it up despite my protests.

"Aw, Kevy, one more go, for old times' sake!" she goads me, in her charming, Australian drawl. "If you don't let me do it now, you know I'll find a way when we're on set. Don't make me hold up filming because your hair is too clean for the camera!" She smiles at me in the mirror, and I submit. Hair and makeup teams are like the bartenders of the set. The actors often get to know them quite intimately because we spend so much time with them throughout the day.

Seal plays softly on the stereo, always a favorite of mine along with Hootie and the Blowfish and the Eagles when I get into Herk mode. Listening to Seal brings back a flood of memories. There were days I thought the show would never end, but, of course, it does. It always does. And I am going to miss it.

I think of the first day I came back to set after falling ill, when this dear friend, Annie, asked me what kind of music I wanted. Because of the size of the production (over seven hundred people worked on the show by now), there were several makeup artists who labored under Annie, but she set the tone and ran the trailer. She controlled the stereo too. We usually had a good rock and roll mix or show tunes. But that first day back I asked simply for quiet.

"Yeah?" she said softly as I sat in her chair.

I looked at my face in the mirror and admitted, to myself as much as to her, "I'm not doing too good, Annie."

She appraised me with a combination of pity and resolve, and then she calmly shooed all the others out of the camper for us to have some peace. She spoke to me in whispers, handling me with kid gloves. It was odd to see her so subdued.

Since then we had worked our way back to an easy, joyful camaraderie. The music now is a good indicator of how far I have come.

Today Annie is bubbling and full of energy, but beneath it all I can tell she is sad. Just as Annie will be looking for a new job, so will most of the rest of the cast and crew. In show business everyone has a kind of gypsy life, moving from place to place, looking for the next paycheck. Landing a series job and keeping it is tough for any of us, and having a series go for seven years is very rare. Together, we had enjoyed building a whole new world. During that span people married (myself included), there were divorces, and babies were born. But every series show eventually finishes, and here I was, at the end of a journey I would never forget.

"How are you today, Kevy?" Annie asks, smiling, her eyes glistening.

"Doin' okay, Annie. Tough day, today." The phrase was getting old, but it seemed to be the only one I could blurt out.

"I know, Kevy, but you're moving on to bigger and better things. Are you excited about the new show?"

"I'd be lying if I said I wasn't. But today . . . the end of an era. This show is all I can think about, honestly. How about you, Annie? What are you going to do without me?" I tease her.

"Aw, you know, find another boyfriend, I guess—someone else to torture!"

We laugh.

"I'm heading back to Australia, I've decided. It's been too long, and these Kiwis are getting under my skin, you know?" she adds, laughing.

We both know she will find work. She is very talented and a joy to be around. She finishes up with an "Okay, big guy! You are good to go. Break a leg!" and pats me on the back.

As I get to the door of the makeup trailer, I look at Annie and thank her for all her hard work. She is about to cry, so I quickly switch gears and tell her the story of my first trip to New Zealand.

In 1992, one year before I booked *Hercules*, I landed a commercial that would film right here in Auckland. It was for Jim Beam Whiskey. I came down for the ten-day shoot very excited to see another part of the world I had never been to before. Immediately I fell in love with the country— its beaches, the bush, the friendliness of its people, and the clean, fresh air. I told myself I would come back to spend more time on both islands. Little did I know that I would book a show called *Hercules* one year later and live a very large chunk of my life here.

The studio we are using today to shoot the final scene ever of *Hercules* is the same studio I shot that Jim Beam commercial in. Things had indeed come full circle.

—

George Lyle, the first assistant director, was in top romantic form when he crafted the schedule for the final shooting episode. He put the ending scene last, which is not often the case. Although this episode is not the final-airing installment (we shot that five weeks ago to accommodate Michael Hurst's schedule with a play he was about to star in and direct), I'm sure that for this last shoot George felt that going out on the endnote was psychologically necessary for us all.

The final scene is a silly one. After helping Autolycus (Bruce Campbell) avoid death by hanging, I help his girlfriend, Luscious Deluxe (Tracy Lord) obtain a bank loan to purchase the club she dances in. When Autolycus, "King of Thieves," hears that banks actually *give* money *out*, he decides on the spot to change careers.

I pat his shoulder, wish him luck, and we share a laugh.

I turn and walk to stage rear, go up three stairs, and turn to the right through a red velvet–curtained archway, leaving the club with a last pensive glance back at my friend.

It's over, I say to myself as I walk offstage. I stop just out of camera range and the sight of my crew. There are a few extras back here— friendly faces who have been with the show for its entire run. They remain quiet. Annie is also back here with us. She gives me a sad smile before I turn my eyes away.

Out of deference to my years playing the illustrious role, Charlie Seibert (yes, the same director who introduced me to my wife, Sam) comes backstage to check that I'm good with the last take. "We're checking the gate, Kevin. Congratulations."

My mind races as I hear George Lyle announce, "That was Bruce Campbell's last shot!" to wild applause.

A spotlight shines on Bruce doing a ridiculous heroic posture dance. The enthusiastic crew spurs him on. Then he says, "But wait" several times until the noise subsides. "But wait, George, who else is wrapped?"

George grabs his head, feigning consternation. "What is his name?"

"What's his name, George? Long hair? Sounds like Bevin, Devin," Bruce continues. I hear someone shout out "Porcules!"

Bruce breaks into the commotion, finally, shouting, "Kevin!"

I'm on the raised platform in the doorway between the red curtains, and a spotlight shines in my eyes to a crescendo of applause. I look around at the cheering crowd, feeling numb. I realize then that while we were shooting our final scene, the entire production office has come to the set to bid the show goodbye. My throat clenches tight and my eyes fill with tears.

I step down to the floor level and look around, applauding them as they clap for me. I had already thanked the crew tearfully at lunch. "Oh! How many speeches am I gonna have to make?" I lament.

The boom mike hovers and the crowd is waiting. My feelings are on high volume. With a shaky voice I tell everyone to come to the party tomorrow, promising to bore them then. As my voice cracks, I yell for Michael Hurst to "take over for me." His long blond locks shorn to near baldness, he is here for the occasion only. I breathe to calm the welling in my throat and manage a big thank you to everyone before I choke some more.

"Hang in there, buddy," shouts a voice from the crew. Others chime in with more encouragement. Annie hands me a tissue, as if that will staunch the torrents of sentiment. I clear my throat again.

"But anyway, I just want to thank everybody here. It's been, uh . . . it's been amazing. God bless." And with a wave of my hands I surrender to my grief and relief all at once. The applause begins immediately and lasts far too long for my comfort. I guess they like to see me cry like a wee baby.

Eric makes his way up, shakes my hand, and we hug. He congratulates the entire cast and crew on completing 111 episodes of *Hercules* and then he pulls out a speech.

"I first met Kevin when I picked him up at the Auckland airport . . ."

"There goes my speech for tomorrow," I tease, evoking a good laugh from everyone.

Eric talks about how we just clicked right away, and he felt like maybe they had really lucked out in casting me. (He lists what he perceives to be my finer attributes as testament.) He turns to me. "Then we pulled up to the hotel, and you said, 'So Eric, what was it that you do on the show, again?' Do you remember that, Kevin?"

In the midst of hearty laughter John Mahaffie shouts out, "And you still haven't told him!"

He answers with hardly a pause, "*I'm* still trying to figure it out!" We all laugh.

Eric finishes with more kind words about me, including Michael Hurst in his heartfelt thanks. Then they present Michael and me with engraved "Official Commemorative *Hercules* Ceremonial Swords." Michael and I immediately pull them out of their velvet pouches for all to see.

Michael shouts, "Hey, wait a minute," noticing that his sword is a good ten inches shorter than mine, but it's all in good humor. The consummate theatrical performer, he brandishes his smaller sword, goading me from on his knees, "Hey, Mister! Just watch it!"

Once Eric is finished presenting our beautiful swords, I see Rob Tapert in the crowd. I walk over to shake his hand and invite him onto the stage.

"I, like Kevin, don't want to give away my speech," he begins, to applause. "This has been the greatest creative experience of my life," Rob continues. "And it wouldn't have been the same without Kevin—from the first time he walked in, and we brought him back seven times," he pauses, just long enough for Eric to sandwich in a good-natured jab: "We were *sure!*"

This gets a good laugh from the audience.

Rob rubs his hands together and continues, "We were sure that he was the person to send down here and torture for seven years if he took seven auditions of torture. So, um, anyways, Kevin, it's been a wonderful experience, and, uh, I couldn't be happier to have had . . . to have an experience with any other actor, so . . . ."

My hand is outstretched and he takes it heartily.

Eric tidies up the presentation with an armed forces saying: "'The difficult is done at once. The impossible takes a little longer.' Seven years ago we gathered together to make what we hoped would be five passable tele-movies, starring a big American hunk with hair extensions," Eric says, pausing for the laugh. "And, yeah, instead, we basically rewrote a chapter in television history. So I would like to thank each and every one of you for making the *Hercules* experience so fun, exciting, and successful for me and for everyone. You've been the best cast and crew a producer could have wished for, and I am, as always, honored to work with you. So thank you all very much, and you guys have a lovely time."

More speeches follow. At one point John Mahaffie jumps up to thank the producers for the special memories and the opportunities that *Hercules* created and offered to New Zealand. "It's been an exquisite experience, and we'll never forget it."

Once it's clear the spotlight is empty, I announce, "I'm just going to go back to my room and have a good cry."

The exquisite experience is over for good.

HERCULES HAS LEFT THE BUILDING

THERE WAS JUST ONE LAST GUY left to part with. Hercules had both created and destroyed me. I guess you never forget your first.

After the big move back to the States, I flew to LA to do some prep work on *Andromeda*. I was focused on making it the best that it could possibly be; with Majel's backing and the Roddenberry name, I felt I had been issued a solemn trust.

In order to be credible as Dylan Hunt, a future space hero, I needed to distance myself from the iconic character that put me on the global scene. I'd made an effort to shed the myth in my mind, but of course, the outside world still identified me with *Hercules*. My next stop was Beverly Hills to get my hair cut short.

It was a strange moment, emotions running high, when I entered the posh salon. I hadn't been this nervous about a haircut since I was a kid, and being greeted by the film crew from *Entertainment Tonight* didn't help. Yep, they deemed this to be a big event and sent a crew to witness the harvesting of my locks! We would be auctioning the shorn hair for charity. They gave me the star treatment, reassuring my raging nerves. When the deed was done and autographs signed, they all said, "See ya' later, Hercules!" as I left. I laughed to myself, realizing that losing him as my identity would not be as easy as trimming my hair.

After that I went to the photographer's studio to shoot publicity stills for *Andromeda*. The studio was an average white loft space in a run-down old 1920s building in Hollywood. It was very LA: stylish, retro, non-chalant. The photographer greeted me at the door.

"Hi. I'm Kevin." I put out my hand to shake. He glanced behind me into the hallway as I shut the door.

Smiling, he shook my hand and said, "Hi. I'm Jim. Uh, where's your entourage?"

I laughed. "Oh, well, I don't . . . it's just me."

"Hercules doesn't need an entourage, eh?" he asked amiably.

I shrugged. "I'm sure the studio has the publicist coming at some point, though."

"I guess it's not like you *need* a bodyguard, is it?" Ha ha ha.

At that moment several people emerged from inside the prep room. "We're here already! Kevin, you're so quiet that we didn't even hear you come in!" I knew the publicist, of course, and also Karen; the remaining introductions were hastily made. Everyone was eager to get started.

"How was it at the salon? I love the new haircut! It completely changes you!" Karen raved. The others agreed and nodded approvingly. It hadn't changed anything, really, but why spoil their party?

The stylist had brought at least ten different outfits to choose from, which were displayed on a rolling clothes rack, but as we all examined the clothes, I yanked out a thin, turtleneck sweater that was black with sparkles. It was some ultramodern type of material.

"This shirt is something I would never wear," I joked. "It's perfect for four thousand years into the future!" The others agreed, so I put it on.

The photographer shot me on a plain white background and was mercifully decisive and expedient. I didn't need to think too much—just follow his directions—which was good because the flashes were sending my brain reeling and I was swiftly getting sick to my stomach.

By the time we finished I was cooked. I limped home to my hotel with a raging migraine and lots of self-doubt. The stress-filled day had been packed and productive, but I wondered, as I did almost every day, how much longer I could keep up the charade of health. My advancements came like honey through a sieve. The eye twitches were gone, the humming in my head had largely abated, and my blind spot, though still there, was something my brain had learned to accept. But I still endured headaches and light sensitivity as well as contended daily with dizziness and nausea. And although working could bring them on, only working distracted me from my worries and suffering.

Hollywood is all show, I thought. The art department would doctor the photos, producing our first *Andromeda* poster, which Tribune would use to sell the show overseas. I would look regal and commanding. *And people believe what they want to believe.* Although I was the one who needed rescuing, I had a new TV show because I could still act like I was saving the world.

In January of 2000 New Orleans hosted the National Association of Television Program Executives Market and Conference, also known as NATPE, the only TV programming market in America that also served the worldwide community. It was a big deal. We were launching the sale of *Andromeda*, hoping buyers from around the world would purchase it for distribution in their own countries. After months of hard work piecing the show together, this would be where all the profit was made. There was a lot at stake.

Tribune wanted me in the booth so I could meet personally with potential buyers. And, of course, they had that poster of me from the chest up, dressed in that vaguely revolutionary futuristic turtleneck. It was straightforward; sales of the show hinged on two things: the Roddenberry name and me.

To end the trip Tribune hosted a large dinner for several hundred clients in one of the hotel ballrooms. At the dinner Tribune chief Dick Askin stood up and gave a short talk about the show and what they were setting out to accomplish (make money), and then he introduced me.

I stood and greeted everyone after being handed the microphone. The glasses stopped clinking and the forks were silenced. All eyes were on me, expectant. Under other circumstances I would have loved this, but with panic attacks always ready to sneak up on me these days, it took all my effort to just appear "normal."

I walked behind my chair and collected my thoughts as best I could. The spotlight helped me focus even as it heightened my anxiety. Performing was always where I felt my best. If I could just get out of my head, so to speak, and into my role, I could even fool myself.

And tonight I did. Although I was clinging to the backrest to keep from falling over, I felt like the star they thought I was, like the prize racehorse to bring them to the finish line. "It's great to be here. Thanks to everyone who made this possible," I grinned and ran down the list of people to be acknowledged. I added, "I've said that I'm going from the past into the future, from Herk to Kirk." I waited for the laughter and comments to die down. "Well, Dick has been joking with me that he wants the same results from this show as *Hercules* was able to deliver during its seven-year run." More laughs. "But I'm not joking. I'm telling you tonight, right here, right now, that *Andromeda* will debut as the number one show in first-run syndication and stay at number one for its *entire* run."

My prediction was met with resounding applause and cheers. I glanced over at Dick, who looked a little shell-shocked. He rebuked me gently with his eyes, as if to say, "Don't write checks you cannot cash, Kevin." But sometimes I just know things, and I was confident—I could feel it. It had Gene Roddenberry's name, and it had me. *Andromeda* would perform well even if I was the only one willing to make that promise. Maybe I threw down that gauntlet for myself, for motivation. If so, it worked. I seized the challenge, wishing only that I knew with as much certainty the future of my health.

⌐‿⌐

Leaving Auckland and *Hercules* behind offered me an opportunity to redefine myself almost entirely, not just cut my hair. I used my time to get settled into a new house in Vegas and catch up with people I hadn't seen for ages. I improved my golf game. I learned how to hold my head so the ball wouldn't disappear, and I trained my brain to expect it and accept it when it did disappear. I worked out at Gold's Gym. I saw my parents a lot. They had moved into a retirement community less than two miles from us. (They said they liked the desert, but I suspect they were anticipating grandchildren.) Basically, I reconnected with myself. It was a period of recalibration and rebirth.

Sam and I made our plans to move to Vancouver, where *Andromeda* would shoot, knowing it was at minimum a two-year commitment.

One evening, while I was studying my lines for the new show, I felt a huge weight of doubt, like mist from a swamp, come and settle on my shoulders. *Andromeda* would *be a hit. It had to be . . . right?* I took a deep breath and looked at Sam in the bed next to me. I envied her, engrossed in her novel. I still was unable to read for long periods, and books remained beyond my reach because of the tight print and my blind spot. Thankfully, I could read scripts enough to memorize dialogue. They had larger print with greater spaces between shorter lines.

I interrupted her. "I hope I can keep up with the schedule up there."

She immediately turned to me and smiled. "Of course you will, darling. You have the twelve-hour door-to-door day in your contract, and on *Herk* you were up to ten. After these few months off for good behavior, you should be fine with the new schedule."

"I know. But what if they expect me to do fight scenes like before?"

"They won't. If they do, you will set them straight."

"Right."

"Kevin," Sam put her book down. "This is just the anxiety talking. It isn't real. There are no issues. You are the star of the new show. You decide what that means. You are the guy who doesn't have to do his own stunts to prove himself."

There were going to be things I wanted to do on the show, I knew—stunts and fights or simple spins, for instance—that were off-limits now. I needed to regulate myself so I wouldn't trip myself up.

"I know. I'm just worried about how they will see me."

"People will treat you the way you teach them to treat you. Your charming, witty personality will win them over," she said with a glint in her eye. She put her hand in mine. It felt reassuring but also insignificant somehow. "Kevin, there are lots of things to worry about, but the new show isn't one of them, okay? You said it yourself. The show's gonna be a hit."

"Yeah, but I'm starting to regret saying that."

"Kevin, if there's one thing I know about you, your bouts of optimism are rare and precious gifts. Don't second-guess yourself now. There's nothing you can do but fulfill it."

She was right. I'd made a prediction, now I had to make it a prophecy. Well, I supposed I was up for the challenge.

Even two and a half years after my strokes I was still testing and discovering boundaries. The good news was that my limitations were improving. The bad news? At some point, I figured, time would play its hand. It was simple math. I had started this ordeal with the brain of an octogenarian. Through rehab and time I had progressed, thankfully, but my recovery would eventually meet my real age. I was just hoping and praying it would be this side of fifty.

In order to get the show bonded (which was partly how a show was funded), the insurance company required their doctor to perform a physical. The physician arrived at my house for the examination. He handed me a bunch of paperwork while he arranged for the blood draw and other tests.

Although *Hercules* had also required exams, production and their doctor already knew my medical history. Now I was concerned that if I divulged my whole history, this new doctor might discover the quaking, vulnerable, brain-impaired man I had become inside. Plus, I really didn't want to talk about it. (That's healthy, right?) But as much as I wanted to, I could not lie. I filled in the entire form and waited for his questions.

"You filled in here that you have suffered a stroke."

Sam was there for moral support. We had discussed how to handle this, and she understood my trepidation. She jumped in, "He had an aneurysm in his shoulder and a few tiny clots somehow shot up into his brain."

"But you're fine now?" he asked offhandedly.

"Yes," I hesitated. "I mean, I'm back to work and everything, so . . . and the doctors have given me a clean bill of health."

"Did they say you were a clotter or give you any explanation for the strokes?"

I fielded this one too. "Well, that's the funny thing. They did all the tests, and I'm definitely *not* a clotter, and because I never took steroids, which was always their second question, they don't have a good explanation. I'm an anomaly, a wild card."

"Oh, well, that's fascinating," he said, pondering.

I smiled, uncomfortable. "Yeah. They keep telling me to play the lottery."

He chuckled amiably. "Maybe they're right. How's your blood pressure?"

"Let's find out." I held out my arm as he cuffed it. Feeling like I had dodged a javelin, I was betting my blood pressure would be rather high, but he made his notes and moved on to finish his exam.

While he packed up his kit, he said, "Take care of yourself. Sorry to hear about your scare. I'm glad for you that it's all resolved and you're back to normal."

"Thank you so much."

Though it was true that I could work a full day by then—I had already proven that on the set of *Hercules*—it was also abundantly clear to me that I was anything but normal. The doctor didn't need to know that, however. Only Sam did.

But it wasn't as if my health issues had magically disappeared. They still haunted me; I simply had learned how to manage them. I am very strong-willed, and although I could not beat my health issues into submission, I often managed to power through, even when they were systematically trying to shut me down.

Of course, sometimes I still gave in too.

DETERMINED

Ardis Sorbo

As a kid, Kevin was a picky eater. If he didn't like what I served for dinner, he would hop on his bike and head for the grocery store with his paper route money to buy Chef Boyardee. He was a doer—if he wanted something done, he did it. He also loved to fish. When fishing season started he would sit on the dock for hours, showing patience I never saw otherwise.

As an adult, Kevin was just as determined. He was a self-made success story.

It was a big shock when Sam phoned us at home in Minnesota to say that Kevin was in the hospital in Los Angeles and that they didn't know what was wrong. Lynn and I were both very upset and offered to come out, but Sam suggested waiting a day or two, just to see. Obviously, as parents, to know our son was in the intensive care unit was difficult. The experience demanded a lot of prayer and faith that things would work out. That time was particularly hard for Lynn, I think, and he even went to our pastor and sent Kevin some books about illness and recovery.

When Cedars let him leave, he shared the whole story: the blood clots and all of that—eleven doctors! We were both concerned and thankful that he was told to rest after they finally diagnosed the strokes. I said, "I'm sorry, Kevin, but your health is the most important thing." I could tell how disappointed he was. He wasn't the usual strong-willed boy I remembered. His illness was a big blow for him and unsettling for us.

While he was recuperating in Vegas, Kevin didn't like to talk very much about how he was doing, but even over the phone line we could tell he wasn't feeling good. We spent a lot of time worrying about him.

Over the years, we visited Kevin in New Zealand a few times. I remembered Kevin's stunt double on the show coming to the trailer to meet us our first visit, saying, "Your son won't let me do anything!" We went to Auckland again after Kevin got sick, and Lynn and I both noticed the huge difference in Kevin's work schedule. Kevin's double was far too busy to complain about being bored anymore!

That Kevin was still able to do the show, knowing how he was feeling and seeing him collapse each day after work, was hard to believe. It was also hard to believe the show could continue with so much less of Kevin. In many ways he wasn't the same young man anymore—except for his unfaltering persistence.

One night while we were there I started choking at the dinner table. When everyone asked me what was wrong, I waved them off and got up quietly to go into the kitchen. I'm not sure why—perhaps I didn't realize how serious it was. But Kevin followed me. He kept asking if I could breathe. Well, I couldn't. So he did the Heimlich on me and out popped a small piece of celery. I took a grateful breath. Thanks to Kevin and his dogged tenacity, I'm alive today. (The next day, though, I asked the set nurse for pain medication because I had such badly bruised ribs!)

This story reminded me of years before, when Kevin was visiting us in Minnesota for the Fourth of July. We were all at a friend's barbecue. Lynn had been lying on a raft in the swimming pool while the large party moved indoors to enjoy a video on TV. Luckily, Kevin went back out to the backyard for something and saw his dad lying on the bottom of the swimming pool. Lynn must have drifted off to sleep and then tumbled into the water—but he didn't know how to swim! Kevin immediately dove in with his clothes on to save him.

So Kevin was our hero long before Hercules.

CINDERELLA

ANDROMEDA OFFERED ME THE OPPORTUNITY to craft a new lifestyle that was both healthier and less intensely work oriented. The first thing I did was give myself plenty of time to get settled and acclimated before starting work. Sam and I arrived in Vancouver, British Columbia, in March of 2000.

Gail, my driver on the show, was a sweet woman who would become a dear friend to us. She picked us up from the airport and drove slowly through the city, introducing us to our new home. The production had rented us a house in Deep Cove, a quiet suburb of Vancouver.

Vancouver was a lush, green, conscientious city, similar to Auckland. Deep Cove had its own distinct personality. Main Street sloped downhill, dead-ending at the cove, which was, uh, quite deep. Boats and kayaks moved silently across the mirrored surface of the black water. Because the tall mountains surrounding it blocked in the clouds, Deep Cove got a lot more rain and gray skies than the rest of the city did. The proud, friendly locals saw that as a practical way to keep unwanted people away. As residents, Sam and I grew to love it there.

Gail turned onto a new street, and Gizmoe sat up, put her paws on the windowsill, and commenced whining and wriggling. When Gail said, "It's just at the end of this hill," I wondered, *how did Giz know we were arriving?* The place had a certain magic, which I took as a good omen.

The next morning Sam and I drove to the studio in Burnaby. We turned in at our address and saw that the building was clearly labeled, "Ackland Warehouses." Sam laughed out loud. "Look! It's like we never left New Zealand almost!" (The airport had also had some major similarities to Auckland, from the welcoming fountain to the indigenous peoples' displays. Clearly, we were in an alternate universe.)

We met everyone in the studio that day, interviewed for a new assistant, and generally got settled in. Although the optimism usually runs high on a new show, this one was guaranteed for forty-four episodes, so to approach this as a long-term commitment was practical, and there was tremendous excitement in the air.

The *Andromeda* sets were almost finished. Touring my spaceship, *The Andromeda*, was surreal: the bridge, where I would be giving orders, the hallways and corridors, my sleeping quarters—all of it immediately took on a life and history for me. My imagination ran like a child in a candy store. The *Eureka Maru*, the clunker ship that would rescue me from my black hole of a grave in the first episode, was a fantastic, creative exercise in engineering and imagination: an old jalopy of a spaceship, patched, mended, and pieced together over decades.

Seeing the ships in person had made the new show more real than any number of scripts could have. I kept telling myself, "I can do this," and now that I had seen the sets, I knew I could. I was euphoric.

When Sam and I got home I collapsed on the couch, wanting to study but knowing I could not focus my eyes enough to accomplish much. Sam made me a hot herbal tea. I never drank hot beverages, but this time I relented. I took the tea and sipped it tentatively. To my surprise, it soothed me. Hot herbal tea would become a welcome new habit we would share at bedtime. My new life had officially begun.

I just glanced at our first call sheet, the schedule for the day's shooting, and knew they couldn't finish my stuff within my twelve-hour stipulation. Each scene for the day was allotted an amount of time, as was hair and makeup for each character, and the lunch break. I knew the scenes, and I understood how much coverage, or different shots (meaning lighting set-ups and camera placements, etc.), each would demand. Let's just say the call sheet was very optimistic. *There's no way.*

Sam pointed out that I had never worked with this director. I certainly didn't relish a showdown or power struggle on my first day, so I observed how filming progressed that morning with apprehension. Maybe he knew some magic way to shoot quickly?

No dice. Shortly after lunch I went to Alan, our director and executive producer, and told him about the time constraints he was facing. He was mystified. "You mean that twelve hours includes the *lunch hour*?" Poor guy. Even if I gave him the lunch hour, something I was not prepared to do, we couldn't make our day. This was a very difficult moment for me because I loved the job and wanted the best show possible. But I also knew that too much exertion would render me useless the next day, and I was worried that I may already be crossing that threshold.

Of course, as was the norm, I was struggling with my illness when we began filming that first day. Certainly, stress played a role in amplifying my issues. My adrenalin was surging, and the rest of my symptoms weren't standing in line for their turn at me, either. Also, to achieve the correct look for the show, our director of photography ordered up a ridiculous amount of smoke to add atmosphere. Smoke makes the scenes and scenery look fantastic on film, but we all complained about breathing it in all day. It was another tax on my system, as were the ship's lights, which strobed and flashed for many of the scenes, with warning bells clanging like lances into my brain. All of these obnoxious external stimuli wreaked havoc on the precarious balance in my head. I desperately wanted to shut my eyes and cover my ears, but that would have been entirely inappropriate (read: unheroic). All I could do was ask politely for them to cut the light effects when we weren't filming, and I stepped outside as often as possible. I was very leery of giving away my health problems, but I was hanging by a thread and I could not afford to stretch any further.

"Alan," I said gently, "I'm sorry, but my contract clearly states twelve hours, door to door."

"Yes," he countered, "but this is our first day."

"I know. All the more reason to make sure we set the tone now and stick to my contract," I answered quietly, nodding. My symptoms were non-negotiable, that much was clear, and Stutz's admonitions to stick to the plan haunted me as well.

There was so much more to be said, but none of it I wanted him to actually know. I had learned a few things from *Hercules*—namely, there were ways a production could work around restrictions when absolutely forced to.

He grumbled a bit, puffed up his chest a little, looked over the call sheet, and then said, "Okay. We'll shoot you out first, then, and pick up that last scene tomorrow, as a one-er."

After that it was never an issue again, although it was the first thing new directors were warned about when working on our show.

It is well known that hour-television is the toughest job in the industry, partly because of its schedule. On a typical television set, filming begins on Monday at around 7 A.M. With reasonable, union-enforced turn-arounds (the time the actor/crew has away from set to regroup and recharge), and given the standard extra-long shoot days, by Friday, filming often runs from 5 P.M. to 7 A.M. Saturday morning. That basically leaves everyone a one-day weekend. It's worse than shift work, where you simply work the odd hours and adjust your sleep schedule accordingly. Changing from normal hours to the late shift each and every week is tremendously taxing on the body.

My unique contract ensured we wrapped every day between 6 and 7 P.M. My twelve-hour door-to-door contract was a brutal demand on the production, but before long many of the crewmembers thanked me for getting them home at a reasonable hour each day and giving them full weekends.

Before my strokes I usually ate lunch with the crew. *Hercules* had been my entire social life, and I enjoyed the camaraderie. After my illness I developed the habit of retiring to my trailer with my lunch for much-needed quiet and time to lie down. This routine carried over on the *Andromeda* set. Although I regretted possibly offending some of my colleagues, I simply had no choice. The long days were tremendously exhausting.

Each morning, from 5:15 to 6:00, I rode a stationary bike to work out my heart, but once I finished shooting, I'd often get in a quick gym session before coming home. These afternoon workouts were a necessary chance to decompress for my addled brain, helping me manage my erratic symptoms. I still had no mastery over my illness—and likely never would—but the workouts gave me an avenue to channel and release my frustration. After dinner with my wife I'd do a little studying and then finish the evening, exhausted, in front of the TV.

Needless to say, this routine was a far cry from the crushing regimen I'd followed before I got sick. My illness had also depleted the muscled physique I'd developed during *Hercules*. At the time I explained to the press and the fans (and even friends) that I had happily shed the extra bulk for my new role. I was amazed at the number of people who approached me to tell me they thought I was bigger. ("I was," I would answer them.) But on a more somber note, I did miss my more muscular body, probably because it was not my choice to drop sizes (it's that control thing again).

Gone were the days of shooting hoops at dusk. I could barely dribble, much less swivel and jump. Now, instead, I had quiet moments with Sam. We'd watch Monday Night Football together, snuggling under a blanket in front of the TV. We'd kayak or bike ride on the weekends. What gradually surfaced in those calm times with Sam were feelings I had never allowed in before—or even knew existed. Relying on other people and realizing that I didn't have to run at full throttle and maintain control at every moment were new concepts for me. And in spite of myself, I gradually began to see beyond the losses and appreciate the rewards of this changed life. I still suffered inexplicable health scares and my symptoms persisted, but I had a routine that was my saving grace, and I had someone else to devote myself to, to share my life with, someone who offered me a focus other than my own frailties. I was well on my way to finding the new me.

NOTHING VENTURED

It is a dark and rainy night, typical of coastal British Columbia in the fall. Sam is driving because, with my eyesight and the rain, I am unable to. It is Saturday, but even after a day of doing very little, my brain is tired from my long workweek.

"Great. Look at this rain. It'll take forever to get there in this." I just don't enjoy going out in public.

Earlier in the day I'd had a tense conversation with Jon, one of my best friends. He was mad at me because I couldn't attend his wedding. It required me to fly across the country, with a connection, drive two hours, and then do the reverse again the following day. "Jon, you don't understand. I really want to come, but I cannot do it." This was, in part, my fault. I had downplayed my illness and limitations, even to good friends, perhaps because of pride or shame—I'm not sure why, exactly. Now, admitting the full extent of my injuries and their effects got me nowhere. It was too late. He was angry, and I am angry now too.

Sam is focused on the road, but she puts her hand on my thigh. "It's not that far. Just relax back, close your eyes, and we'll be there before you know it."

"Tell me again why we are doing this? We don't even know these people. He's bringing his wife?" We are driving in the downpour to a fish restaurant way across town for dinner with someone we met last spring on an airplane.

"He's in town with her. I think they are going on an Alaskan cruise. He was very nice and funny when we met him, remember? I thought it would be fun. He is also a furniture connection for us."

Sam thinks we should design a furniture collection—for fun. "Right, the furniture guy. But really, is this going to be worth it?" I am thinking of what my brain's reaction might be tomorrow.

"It's too late to cancel now. Although I admit I wonder what they are really like. He rides a Harley, you know? And apparently they are really into bowling."

"That's promising. I mean, we really have no idea who these people are. I don't get why we have to do this, in weather like this, especially."

"Don't worry. Once we get out of Deep Cove, it'll probably clear up a bit, and as for the evening, well, it's an adventure."

Sam craves the social stuff. She probably needs to get out on the town a bit and get this out of her system. I'm lucky we are both homebodies for the most part, but I guess even that can get old. I look at her, thinking she is truly the only one who comes close to understanding me.

We get to the restaurant, and the maître d' shows us to our table, explaining that the other couple arrived early but left to watch the hockey game in the bar across the street. *Okay*, I think, *they like hockey. That gives us something in common.*

I glance at Sam, and she has an incredulous expression on her face. "What if she shows up in a muumuu and curlers?" she giggles. I'm thinking it might not be such a joke.

We sit down and look at our menus. "Listen Sam, when dinner is done, I just want to get back home, okay? Please let's not just hang out afterwards."

A smiling hostess approaches the table, followed by our dinner companion, Bill, who is wearing khaki shorts that are completely incongruous with the outside weather. "I didn't know it was goin' to rain like this. All I packed were shorts!" He is self-effacing and has a paunch, something the tropical Hawaiian shirt is obviously meant to conceal. His accent is a light, nasally southern drawl, and there is a perpetual twinkle in his eye. "Joann'll be here soon, but she wanted to see if they would score another goal before the end of the second period." We start an easy conversation about the inclement weather, and I casually scan the incoming guests, noticing an attractive, lean woman in a black suit. *That can't be her*, I think, but Bill stands up and introduces his beautiful wife, Joann.

Dinner is served. Bill reveals this is the second marriage for them both—to each other. "She divorced me and then decided that she couldn't live without me, so I agreed to take her back," he explains facetiously. Bill and Joann have an easy rapport and well-rehearsed stories that are tremendously entertaining.

"When I crashed the scooter, I managed to ensure that I landed just under Joann, to break her fall." He gestures with one hand landing gently on top of the other.

"*So* gentlemanly!" Joann interjects sarcastically.

"Then *she refused* to get back on the scooter with me!" he narrates, feigning bafflement at her reluctance, as she shakes her head in utter disagreement. "So I drove the entire way back on my broken scooter, my clothes ripped and bloody from the wreck, to get her some help."

Joann jumps in, in her delicate deadpan drawl, "To get me a ride home, you mean!"

"Whatever she wanted was my thinking," he says, the epitome of gallantry. "So the whole way back—must've been at least five miles—the cars coming toward me were shouting things at me I couldn't understand. I thought, jeesh, can't they see I'm in bad shape? Why are they just yelling at me the whole time? So I started giving them the finger and shouting at them unkindly as they came at me." Bill waves a fist in the air for emphasis.

Joann reaches up to bring his hand down, saying, "It wasn't 'til he got to the rental place that he found out the island road only goes one way!"

On the drive home Sam is beaming. I too am still smiling from the laughs we shared with our new friends. It was the most fun I'd had in a long time, actually. I realize that I could stand to broaden my horizons every now and then, that if I don't feel like doing something, maybe it is something I need to do anyway.

I reach over and grab Sam's hand.

A few weeks later Sam leads me down the rocky steps to the diminutive doorway of a half-underground unit. We stand outside on a porch area, overgrown with the dense foliage of a rain-soaked land. Sam knocks, and the door immediately opens on a small radiant woman, Lee. She has wild black hair with an impressive white streak.

"Kevin, Sam told me a lot about you. I am so pleased to meet you." She graciously invites us in. "My goodness, you are really tall! I have to admit, I am a big fan. I watched *Hercules* all the time."

The ceilings in her little clinic are less than seven feet, making me feel like a giant. "Fi, fie, fo, fum!" I say, laughing.

"I know, it's built for pygmies, but it's fine for me!" she says, ushering me into her treatment room. She has a soft, supple voice like a warm Hawaiian breeze.

"Let's get you lying down before you knock your head. Watch the doorway! There's a gown on the bed there. Please put that on." I duck into a tiny white room with a hospital bed, some wall cabinetry, and a high window that looks into foliage. A low, shaded lamp softens the claustrophobic feeling in the room only a little.

After I change into the hospital gown, careful not to hit anything, and open the door for them, I lie on the bed. Lee asks, "Would you like Sam to stay in the room?"

"Sure." Sam quietly takes a chair in the corner. She recently met Lee at a Christmas party and insisted that I give her acupuncture a try, just to see if we can knock my symptoms off-balance enough to readjust them, maybe even cure them somehow. It's a ridiculous hail Mary–type of play, but my recovery seems to have plateaued and I'm out of options, so I am willing (again) to try something new.

We carefully disclose the source of my issues. Lee takes it all in with a sigh and a smile. She takes my pulse with her fingers on first one wrist and then the other. She nods and grunts—in either disapproval or acceptance, I am not sure which.

She settles on a course of action for her needles and begins flitting around me with a cotton ball soaked in alcohol, swabbing me in various areas—the insides of my knees, my neck, my wrists, and, of course, my left arm. As she taps a thin needle into my flesh at my ankle, I yelp. She looks concerned. "It is highly unusual for my patients to feel the needles going in," she states, matter-of-factly. Well, I felt that one, along with every one after that. The session is very uncomfortable, but I do feel different when she finishes about an hour later.

Sam and I leave and get in our car. Sam sits there for a moment before starting the engine.

"What is it?" I ask her.

"She knows," she answers.

"What?" I am stupefied. "Why did you tell her?"

"I didn't tell her anything. I just got a feeling, the way she shook my hand goodbye. She held it just a bit too long. I think she knows, somehow."

We had found out two days before that Sam was pregnant. Although we were excited and overjoyed, we had agreed not to tell anyone for three months. "Don't be ridiculous, Sam, she's not a witch. She can't know," I say, unconvinced. "I'm glad you didn't tell her though," I smile. "I like that it's our little secret for now." I reach over to grab her hand, pulling it to my lips.

About a week later I am on break in the desert when my phone rings. It's Lee, calling to follow up on how I am doing after our first treatment. I believe she helped me, I tell her. Then she asks me, "And how is Sam doing? I got the distinct impression that she was pregnant when I saw you guys here . . ."

A chill runs through me, but I answer her, "Yes, she's fine. She knew you knew, by the way."

Lee's sparkling laugh makes me think of Glenda, the good witch.

Blasting out of nowhere, Kevin Sorbo made a triumphant transition from swap to ship with the debut of Tribune's weekly hour, Gene Roddenberry's Andromeda *this season.*

—Electronic Media*

The last *Hercules* episode aired in January of 2000. *Andromeda* debuted in October, pulling in a 4.3 rating and soundly thrashing all competition for the number-one spot in first-run syndication. My prediction at NATPE had been vindicated! Not since *Hercules's* spin-off, *Xena*, which benefitted from the *Hercules* action hour as lead-in, had a syndicated show debuted over a 4 rating, and the only other show to do it before that was when *Hercules* debuted!

My manager called to deliver the incredible news: These accomplishments soundly placed me third on Electronic Media's list of "Most Bankable On-air Personalities in Syndication" after Regis Philbin and Oprah (not bad company—though sadly, I was not in their pay scale!).

I had made good on my boast at the NATPE dinner. I had somehow beaten the odds and landed on top. I had proven to the world and, more importantly, to myself, that I was still a valuable player, capable of great things. It was a proud moment when my manager told me about the fantastic article, and in addition to solidifying my self-respect and credibility again, it also did something more than that.

Now that the goal was fulfilled, I could appreciate the superficial victory it represented. Nothing had changed—nothing. Sure, I was a great big TV star again, but I was still the same old guy with the same old migraines and health challenges. Life was the same. I couldn't decide whether to laugh or cry.

Dr. Stutz had said that accepting and integrating the shadow version of myself would make me a better actor. I decided I had nothing more to lose. I let Mr. Shadow onto the set. He began to inform my perform-

---

*"You Can Take It to the Bank" by Chris Pursell; *Electronic Media;* January 15, 2001; Crain Communications Inc.

ances, and through that odd type of therapy, I started to accept him. When I felt weak, I embraced it. I acted through it instead of pretending it wasn't there. If a throbbing head frustrated me, I stopped fighting it and let my character have a headache; I let anger and irritation have their way in the scene, and I was surprised to find them useful. I used the emotions my illness evoked as fodder for the relationship I was portraying on screen. Sam commented to me that she thought my performances were becoming more compelling to watch. At last I began to find contentment within the limitations my illness imposed.

MAGIC

IN 1990 LYNN SWANN INVITED ME to golf at a prestigious golf club in LA. When I got to the beautiful clubhouse on Pico Boulevard I discovered that I would be golfing with Sidney Poitier. I had always admired his superb acting, and now I had the chance to tell him in person.

The introductions made, we started on our round, hitting easy drives down the first fairway. Mr. Poitier walked beside me in silence on the soft green carpet for a few minutes. Nervous and intimidated, I was trying to find the words to start a conversation when he said, "Kevin, golf . . . represents . . . self," and he put his hand gently on my shoulder for emphasis. He had a seeming divine authority that left me speechless. I pondered his words as he walked off toward his ball. That was all he needed to say. It was truth and it was poetry, and it made me grin.

Golf is one of the most frustrating of games, but a single well-struck golf shot was all it took to hook me so many years ago. I was a barefoot, shirtless kid, hitting the links where my dad moonlighted as manager of Lakeview Public Golf Course, when I fell in love with the game. The first time I hit the ball perfectly, it flew beautifully far away, and I was captivated. I needed to do it again . . . and again . . . and again! A good golf shot has a graceful elegance, and the sweet, pure contact with the clubface resonates up the arms, inducing a high that cannot be resisted.

Golf became my therapy immediately, although as a young kid I didn't really need it, as such. Over the years my love affair with the game developed into my release, my comfort, and my distraction. Stamina is the only limitation for a golf addict like myself. I would happily play more than thirty-six holes on any given day, but at four and a half hours, a full round of eighteen holes is usually enough to satisfy and tire even the most intrepid golfers. Before I got sick I would often hit the links as soon as the course opened in the morning, which meant I was the only one out there for at least that first fifteen minutes. This virtually ensured that, with no one ahead of me, I could finish a full round in less than three hours if I walked. (I would do eighteen on a cart in an hour and a half.) Yep . . . get out of my way—I play fast! First off the tee was a reasonable solution for my impatience. It also helped improve my game.

Of course, when I got sick, my game vanished, just like a ball in the upper right quadrant of my sight. I still loved the game, but with my balance compromised, just standing still over a golf ball became an enormous challenge. I battled back. I needed to play, and frankly, with fewer distractions outdoors, as it required only walking, I saw golf as therapeutic on two levels.

The first time I played, about nine weeks into my recovery, I shot a 97—for nine holes. Typically, I would shoot a 76 or 78 for a full 18. It was embarrassing and demoralizing. At that time I never once imagined that my reprieve might come on a golf course.

~

It is February of 2001. The scene is the AT&T Pro-Am at Pebble Beach. Though the celebrity committee has invited me for years running, I never had a break in my *Hercules* schedule to allow me to go. With *Hercules* wrapped now, finally, sick or healthy, I am determined to attend.

For me this is the Holy Grail of golf: the spectacular Pebble Beach Golf Course, which lyrically winds its way over the breathtaking Monterey Peninsula's oceanside cliffs and offers golfers from all over the world a bona fide Mecca for play. I am very excited and nervous. Although I lead a basically normal life now, I combat my ever-present symptoms daily. The extra nerves for this tournament might just sucker-punch me.

I don't care. Whatever happens, I am determined to power through somehow.

Checking in at the hotel, I feel pretty good. I figure I must be high on the idea of finally participating in the AT&T, so I play it safe, ordering in a steak and going to bed early. Sam, three months pregnant, will join me in two days, so for now I'm on my own.

In the morning, it's amazing. I still feel great. The humming in my head has inexplicably quieted. I am so stoked about playing that I don't even pause to consider whether this is a good or bad sign. I welcome the inner peace, prepare my clubs, and head downstairs for a healthy breakfast.

I run into Leslie Nielsen, who has a whoopee cushion with him (as always). Kevin Costner, the consummate gentleman, pats me on the back and wishes me luck. I see many of my old golfing pals at the buffet: Billy Andrade, Mark O'Meara, and Brad Faxon are among them. It feels really cool that they are happy to see me too. They are my heroes, and being able to chat with them, almost like old friends, is fantastic. Because I haven't seen most of these guys in a very long time, we catch up a bit on what's happening in their lives and they also ask about my "health scare."

"It's all good," I say easily. I don't want to be a downer. I don't want to admit any health issues, and frankly, I am feeling pretty great right now. Unsurprisingly, the lessening of my symptoms proves to be a true boost to my morale and confidence.

My playing partner is pro-golfer John Cook, and we are paired with Notah Begay and Craig T. Nelson. I've already met John at other tournaments, and Notah is an easygoing pro who played at Stanford with Tiger Woods. I discover Craig is a very relaxed, fun guy. He will turn out to be a good friend. I figure I need to conserve all my energy for the golf, not conversation, so I keep a low profile.

On the second day of competition we are playing the world famous Pebble Beach Golf Course. It is a sunny, windy, cloudy, rainy, sunny, three-seasons-in-one-day kind of weather. Impervious, I say a prayer of thanks for being invited to such an amazing place.

Irish golf commentator and former European and PGA tour pro David Feherty follows our group as we progress down fairways lined with enthusiastic yet always polite spectators. He interviews Craig and me, but he's here for Notah, who is currently in second place.

Yesterday was rained out, so today, Saturday, the crowds are even bigger than expected. I sign several autographs between each hole. Fans offer me all kinds of encouragement.

In spite of putting on rain gear and stripping it off repeatedly, I am playing very well: only three over par coming into the last four holes. On the par-five fifteenth, a sharp dogleg to the right, I swing my driver and send my golf ball screaming down the center of the fairway. It is a perfectly struck ball, making me feel stupendous. Of course, this is particularly true because millions on TV witness it alongside me. It may sound juvenile, but I briefly feel like a hero again.

Oddly, there is no tingling or pain in my arm as well as no nausea. The incessant humming is quieted and the dizziness has reduced to an all-time low. My blind spot is practically the only vestige of my crisis. I am mysteriously renewed and euphoric.

My caddy and I approach the ball on the fairway, and he judges the distance to be about 238 yards to the pin, but it's playing more like 260 to the elevated green. This is one of the toughest par fives on the tour. I ask him for my three-wood, line up my shot with a grin, and tell him I am going for it, instead of playing it safe. This is too much fun.

I nail the shot, though it gets a bad kick. Like I said, a hard green to hit, and even though I am pin high, I have a thirty-yard shot now to a pin that offers no green to work with—in other words, a tough shot.

After my three-wood shot, Feherty exclaims on camera, "This bloody Hercules is playing out of his bloody gourd!"

I turn back to him and give him a mischievous smile. He is absolutely right.

I line up my next shot, next to the large crowd, hitting a beautiful lob wedge to within inches of the hole for a birdie! That day I turn in an impressive (for me) two-over-par seventy-four.

The entire two and a half years since my strokes, my illness has been a full-time, ever-present guessing game. For this one magical week in

Monterey, it all but disappears. Was it the intense focus on the game in an on-camera pressure situation that worked some magic? Was it just something I ate or something I breathed on the ocean breezes? I'll never know.

Regardless, I am thankful to get even a brief taste of normal again, the sort of basic brain function that is so easy to take for granted in the rush of a demanding workweek and busy schedule. Later, I am also grateful that I have no apparent repercussions from the week, although my symptoms return in full force on the plane ride home. I sit in my narrow, commuter-plane seat, feeling the dizziness start on takeoff. As we climb, the familiar head rush and the thrum of my old companion rejoin me, and I wonder, *More? Really? Okay, then, here we go again.*

I shrug and turn my thoughts back to my Pebble Beach tournament score of seventy-four. I *was* out of my gourd, in a nearly literal sense. My reprieve fills me with hope—hope that a better life still lies ahead.

GRACE

AT THE END OF *Hercules* season one, after trying out a hideous, ten-foot, beast-creature for the part of Ares, the writers crafted a new, human-like god of war. The move was brilliant, particularly because of the casting. The producers chose a local actor named Kevin Smith. Kevin's dark good looks, athletic body, and wicked sense of humor were perfect to play the part of Hercules's dashing, evil half-brother, and Ares became our most beloved villain.

On the personal side Kevin and I made fast friends. He was a dedicated actor with quick-witted comedic timing and a relaxed, jovial presence on the set—a class act. We staged epic fight scenes together and laughed through the sweat when they were finished. And it didn't hurt that we both shared a fondness for golf. We hit the course on a regular basis, and had we known at the time that reality TV was coming down the pipe, we would have filmed our golfing days because they were hilarious.

I nicknamed Kevin "Monkey Boy." He was rarely in the fairway, seemingly preferring the trees and rough for the more challenging golf shots they offered. He also had a lively temper, which, combined with his humor, made the "long walk spoiled" even longer—but a lot funnier. Kevin regularly broke clubs and dropped to the ground for push-ups to cool his temper after bad shots.

The autumn after *Hercules* wrapped filming for good, Rob Tapert asked me to return to New Zealand to guest star on *Xena*. While I was down there I scheduled another round of golf with Kevin Smith and Ge-off Dolan. We enjoyed the day on my former golf course, Titarangi, a lush, well-designed track that I loved. It was much like old times and a nice trip down memory lane for me. Kevin shanked his ball left and right, and he teased Geoff and me about our shots (as if he had any right to comment). We laughed a lot.

That night we attended Kevin's weekly Improv Sports Theatre group at a local restaurant, where he and other talented actors improvised scenes for exercise and fun. Kevin was in rare form. There is a Hollywood phrase for when an actor feels like someone got a part (or parts) out from under him: "He has my career." Well, in all modesty, I had Kevin's career. He really deserved big Hollywood stardom, and there was nothing standing in his way but fate. I sat in my seat nursing a nonalcoholic beer and watching him perform, being thoroughly entertained.

When he dropped me at the hotel and said good night, I answered, "Good night, mate. I'll see you in Hollywood." I was referring to his solid gold future.

I got the phone call from Michael Hurst. After finishing filming a movie in China, Kevin Smith had fallen several stories off some sort of scaffolding. He had immediately slipped into a coma and was being treated in a hospital ICU in China.

I was dumbfounded. This did not fit with my reality. Kevin was a vibrant personality and a truly gifted performer, not some guy lying under a sheet in a hospital room. I hated picturing him there; visions of my own struggle came flooding back to me. It took a few days for the truth to sink in.

Michael called me and e-mailed every day with updates on Kevin's status, which did not change until he died, ten days later. When Michael called to tell me Kevin had passed away, we both broke down and cried openly on the phone. I knew the call was going to come, but I didn't want to hear it. I hung up the phone and went to the gym to work out my anger. The bench press barely made a dent, but yelling helped a little, and my headache afterward was totally worth it.

I tried in vain to make sense of the tragedy. Kevin was on the brink of enormous success. After China he had been scheduled to play in a big

Bruce Willis movie, to add to his growing list of film credits. He was booked on the international stage and ready to make the move to Hollywood.

Not anymore.

Kevin died in 2002 at the age of thirty-eight, the same age I was when I had had my own brush with death and at a similar point in his career. What meaning was there in this bit of coincidence? He died of a head injury, but I somehow had survived three blood bullets to my brain. *He has my death,* I thought. *There, but for the grace of God go I.* I thought about the last time I saw him, outside my hotel in Auckland, and I grieved the great loss his death represented. I wondered about his widow and three young boys, and then I cried some more.

A few years after his passing I traveled back to New Zealand. Geoff Dolan graciously took me to Kevin's grave so I could have some kind of closure. We sat next to his tombstone and toasted Mr. Smith with a couple of beers. We talked about old times, golf, and improv, but mostly we sat in silence. Fans and friends had come by, leaving bottles of his favorite beer and flowers to pay homage to a man who died too young, with too much left to do. Quietly, slowly, I said a prayer and begged for some answers.

I struggled to find some meaning in all of it, but I did not succeed. Because there is a God I am convinced there is a reason, but my lesson from this was that I was very lucky.

And life is short. It really is.

SMALL MIRACLES

AT ABOUT FOUR O'CLOCK on a sweltering August afternoon I am getting in my daily cardio on the stair machine when Sam, about fifty-five pounds heavier than when I first met her, lumbers upstairs and stands watching me, smiling. I smile back at her, briefly flashing to our whale-watching trip on a friend's boat a few weeks earlier. I had pointed at her and shouted, jokingly, "Oh, look! It's *Samu!*" Sam was good-natured about her pregnancy, so that didn't land me in the doghouse, luckily.

"I thought you were going for a nap?" I ask her as I work the machine.

She shrugs. "I couldn't fall asleep. How much longer do you have on that thing?"

Damn, she carries that extra weight well. From behind, you cannot tell she is pregnant, and she has that *glow* in her face.

I look down at the readout. Fifteen minutes have elapsed.

"About twenty minutes," I answer nonchalantly, thinking I would move to free weights after this.

"Um, no, you don't." She smiles sweetly and serenely at me. "My water broke. We need to go to the hospital now to have a baby." She says it so calmly. I freeze, taking in the news.

I am suddenly, completely refocused. I jump down from the stair-stepper and take off running to grab all the things we had decided months ago we needed at the hospital. Where the heck are they? Not packed in a bag, ready to go, of course. She is still two weeks from her due date.

My childhood buddy Jon and his wife are visiting, sitting in the family room when we enter to give them the news. Sam has my hand, and she is visibly shaking. Her excitement is contagious, and my voice trembles as I explain where we are headed.

The hospital is hurry-up-and-wait. The nurses tell us she is not dilated at all, so we should just go for a long walk. It is August in Vegas. Outside, the 104-degree heat envelops us as we stroll the hospital parking lot. Not the most romantic place to be, with the sounds of traffic and the breeze carrying wafts of car exhaust, but Sam is not about to drive anywhere.

Eight laps around the hospital later, we go back into the L&D area for another checkup. No change. They hook Sam up to some drugs and tell us she will likely deliver first thing in the morning.

"You should go home and get some rest." Sam suggests.

"What? No. I'll stay here with you."

"Kevy, it's going to be a long night. I'd rather you got your rest so you'll be more useful tomorrow," she smiles.

"Very funny, but I don't want to leave you here alone."

"Let me call Gina. I'll see if she can come, okay? There is just no reason you should lose sleep for this right now. Plus, your friends are still at the house. I'll be sure to call you if anything changes, but otherwise, just plan to come first thing in the morning, 'kay? I love you."

"Love you more," I say, relenting. It was an attack on my ego, but these days I recognize even my smallest limitations and accept them more readily.

After a fitful night I am back the following morning. "You missed the whole thing!" Sam teases me, then succumbs to a very painful contraction.

Sam has still not dilated, and she finally consents to an epidural in preparation for the impending C-section. That expertly placed needle does the trick—no cesarean necessary. About an hour (and only five pushes) later, Braeden Cooper Sorbo comes into the world at 1:39 P.M.

I have just witnessed the birth of my first child.

Ecstatic tears flow down my face. Everything slows down. I am so overwhelmed with emotions I have never felt before: instantaneous love for a child I don't know yet, an urge to protect him, intense gratitude for being part of a miracle. My focus is entirely fixed on this tiny, wrinkled, strange-looking body. He is the most beautiful thing I have ever seen. The sensation of fatherhood engulfs me. If pride is a sin then I am—and remain to this day—guilty. Braeden's birth is by far my proudest moment. My life immediately becomes his.

Almost as important to me, Mom and Dad are also there to greet their new grandchild into this world. They wait in the room named for that purpose. (Dad told me that he didn't witness the actual births of his five children, and he wasn't going to start now—and he calls himself a biology teacher!)

My son's entrance into the world represents a rebirth for me: a new, greater, and more challenging role than any mythical or science fictional character, one that demands not just my heart but also my soul. My innocent, helpless son requires a love and devotion from me that is entirely selfless, while my life before now was more introverted than I care to admit.

Braeden has unwittingly given me another glimpse of God—the supreme poet, the balancer of life—and He is truly generous. I send Him my prayers and thanks for letting me experience this day.

⌁

My new son finally justified my illness-forced domesticity. I was no longer staying home in the evening because I couldn't afford to tax my brain; I was enjoying my son, spending time with him and caring for him.

For *Andromeda*'s second season, Sam and I had moved into a small, quaint home in Dunbar, an older suburb of Vancouver with grid streets and heritage-style houses on gentle slopes, as well as parks in every direction. Each day I happily returned home from filming to Braeden's wide smile and pumping fists, his uncontainable excitement. I looked forward to our long evening walks with the Baby Björn or stroller.

Sam also often brought Braeden down to set for lunch on her way somewhere, and we would play for a few minutes in my camper. She was more vigilant with my rest periods than I was, and she would conveniently arrange to visit with other crewmembers while I caught my necessary midday lie-down. I had learned to manage my symptoms and accept them. Only rarely did they completely sideswipe me, although my migraines were still an aggravation, challenging me in increasingly perplexing ways.

I eventually sought out a highly recommended neurologist at Vancouver General, who was very nice but offered me no solution or even advice. I found it fascinating—and frustrating—that each time I related my story, the doctor's inevitable reaction would be amazement, empathy, and . . . impotence. I was beyond the books and the journals. It was like I was working my way through a dense rain forest without a machete, and the guides, behind me, were offering me bubble gum.

As I found ways to cope with and accept my issues, the *why* of it all faded into the background. Sam and I were in bed one night and I mentioned that I never got the answer to *why?*

She studied me for a moment and said, "Well, if it's any consolation, you know, if you hadn't gotten sick, I don't know if we would have lasted."

She took me completely off guard and I pulled back in disbelief. "What? What do you mean by that?"

"I'm just saying that you were speeding through life, a hundred miles an hour. You didn't really have time for me. It was my job to fit into your life if I wanted to be with you. I went to the gym, I learned to golf. If I wanted to spend time with you, well, we had to do what you planned to do."

"Listen, I was working really hard . . ."

"I'm not saying it was right or wrong, Kevin. I'm not criticizing. I'm just stating fact. The gym and golf were good for me, and I liked doing them with you—for you."

"Yes, they were. Plus, you got into great shape," I said proudly.

She continued, "But now, with our baby, he needs you even more than I do, and you need to be with him, and with your old schedule, I don't know if that would have happened. And to be perfectly honest, I don't know how long I would have put up with just tagging along on your hectic, packed life."

How could I answer her?

"I mean, it did almost kill you," she concluded.

My life had been pretty amazing—flying all over the world, fame, money, success. It would have been a fantastic ride. Then again, add a baby into that mix and I wasn't exactly sure what would have come out of it. Would I have taken the time to really appreciate that gift?

"Kevin, God tapped you on the shoulder and told you to slow down. I think you are lucky to be alive." She kissed me goodnight and arranged her pillows as she laid her head down. "And I'm lucky too."

Why? was a bogus question, a distraction. Someday, it might become perfectly clear, but it would not matter in the end. I turned out the light while I pondered this new perspective.

Our little boy was the reason I rushed home each night. I relished our evening walks to the park with him in the stroller. Every new thing he learned excited me. He stole focus from my demons, making me smile even when I was feeling awful.

When he was just over a year old we were on hiatus in Henderson, and we found out Sam was pregnant again. The news was doubly exciting, though, and we rushed to my parent's house to share it.

"Dad, what's your favorite baseball team?"

"The Minnesota Twins, why?"

"Because we just came from Sam's ultrasound."

"Oh, for heavenly days!" My mom was quick-witted and immediately got my hint. "Lynn, they are expecting twins!"

"Oh, ho, ho! No kidding? That's wonderful! That's just wonderful news!" Dad hugged Sam. I hugged my mom.

Sam beamed at me. "And I'll predict right here and now that they will come out boy—then girl!"

"Well, when the first one was a boy, I was kind of surprised, but now, I'm going to buy into the whole prophetic thing," I laughed.

"Oh, sweetie, you know you make your own destiny. We have an agreement on two boys and then a girl," she explained to my parents.

"I remember!" Mom insisted. My parents were truly overjoyed to be coming into more grandchildren.

Preparing to add substantially to our family was exciting, and we shared our good news with many friends over the following few months.

⌐‿⌐

I had seen Lee, the acupuncturist/witch/friend, many times over those first few years. Between the needles and some other nonmedical treatments, like sweat baths in peat and herb-infused enemas, I had actually improved. Eventually Lee talked me into doing a full, intensive week of therapy. There was no way I could manage that during my shooting schedule, so we planned a trip for her to visit us in Las Vegas during a hiatus from the show.

Lee arrived at our house, surprised by Gizmoe, who met her, barking, at the door. She seemed overwhelmed and distant, but she explained simply that she had no idea we had a dog and wasn't really partial to small canines. (Gizmoe quickly won her over.) She unpacked her things in our guest room and we enjoyed a nice dinner together, sharing our great news that Sam was thirteen weeks along on babies two and three.

The next day Sam went off to her doctor's appointment while Lee started me off with an herbal enema, needles, and some smoldering stick to heat the needles, which would in turn affect the way they worked. I cannot explain how these ancient Chinese treatments are supposed to operate, but I trusted her and committed to being her guinea pig for the next week. After the first treatment was over I went out to run some errands. Then I came home to a somber household.

Sam was in bed, despondent.

"What's wrong, honey?" I approached the bed and stroked her cheek. This was completely out of character for Sam; I'd never seen her like this.

For several moments she literally could not produce the words.

"I lost them!" she finally blurted.

"Lost what? Hmm? Whatever it is . . ." And then my heart nearly stopped. I *knew* then. "What? What happened?" My skin was suddenly cold and clammy, my breath stilled. How could they be gone, these two little lives that would complete our family? "Tell me—what happened?"

"Nothing happened. They 'failed to thrive.' That's what they call it. They stopped living is all. There's no heartbeat. They're gone. I . . ." she took a ragged breath. "I asked them to . . . to show me. I had to see. They didn't want to, but . . . I made them *show* me. I saw the, uh, ultrasound. There were the little . . . they didn't have any heartbeats anymore. Not anything."

I held her and felt her sobbing in my chest. I wanted to crawl into a cave, to punch something, to yell at the top of my lungs. "She cried for me, you know? The doctor, she was so upset, she cried. I couldn't—I didn't cry, at first. I didn't believe it. When I first went in I told them I felt great, and they said that I had lost weight, and I said it didn't matter because I was sure everything would be fine. I'm such an idiot."

"Wait a minute, Sam, there's nothing you could have done. There's nothing different you could have done. This just is . . . well, it just is."

"Yeah, but it changes everything now. I was so certain, you know?"

Yes, I knew exactly. Sam had this optimistic attitude that pervaded her entire psyche. While I sometimes found it annoying, I envied her as well. She assumed the twins would be part of the family we had envisioned on our first date—we both did—but now fate had proved her wrong. I felt awful: first from the loss of the babies to come, and second, I had the worried feeling I was not on fate's winning team anymore. Maybe my lucky streak was, in fact, coming to an end. I knew that thinking of life in those terms was ridiculous, but there was a romantic side of me that clung to the idea that things in life happen for a reason. The reasons had now become more sinister, apparently.

Over the next week Lee treated me and also ministered to Sam in her grief, stating matter-of-factly, "This is why I came now and not before." I believe her apparent negative reaction to Gizmoe when she arrived was to cover her realization, upon first seeing Sam, that we had already lost the babies.

Although the sense of loss was still palpable, after a few days life had almost the appearance of back to normal. After all, Sam had a toddler to chase.

Five years after my strokes I was still making small improvements on a long road that no doctor had charted. They had been wrong about their initial three- to eight-month recovery, and I was getting stronger every day. I kept reminding myself just that.

As a result of Lee's treatments, however, I improved drastically. Her odd concoctions and machinations with needles, smoke, and herbs somehow managed to knock my illness around enough for me to feel more in charge. My headaches were less severe and more manageable. My dizziness somehow seemed less formidable. Lee taught Sam how to apply tiny ball magnets on small square pieces of tape to my ears. The ears are very sensitive. (Try wearing sunglasses that hit your ear the wrong way and you will appreciate very quickly how strongly the outer ear reacts to stimuli.) Maybe these magnets simply distracted me, but regardless, I felt less dizzy and nauseated. I had found a homeopathic therapy for many of my issues. Lee gave me the edge I needed to feel effective against the enemy I was fighting. My symptoms won the occasional battle, but when I returned to work later that spring, it was with a renewed confidence and a lighter step.

That summer Sam became pregnant again, but my heartbreak over the loss of my children endured for a long, long time. I kept it buried inside, but the anger and the hurt lived on.

I still had a lot to learn.

Braeden's nursery was sweet and cozy: lavender walls, a white crib, and blowing curtains on a window overlooking our tree-lined suburban street. Every evening, while the sun lazily set on another day, we sat in a rocker near the window, reading books before I lay Braeden gently down to sleep. Because I worked on the set most days, his bedtime routine was all mine and I cherished it. He too loved our quiet time together, always clamoring for more snuggling or another hug and, more importantly, another laugh. His laugh at my voices as I read books to him made me smile the biggest smile you can imagine.

At the end of each reading time I would pick up my son, carry him over to his crib, and, with a monster hug and kiss, lay him down and maybe sing him a song or two. I had to creep out of the room, leaving the door with its mandatory crack of light coming through. He loved that crack of light . . . a child's comfort.

And now we had another baby boy on the way. Sam had set up the bedroom across the hall with a new race-car bed, perfect for a toddler. We decided to move Braeden in advance of the baby's arrival so he wouldn't "blame" the baby for displacing him. I remember the first night I read to Braeden in his new room and tucked him into his fantastic new bed. He was very excited. I kissed him goodnight and walked slowly to my bedroom down the hall.

I got into bed with my script, ready to review my lines for the next day. Sam was beside me, reading.

I just sat there, unable to focus. Sam glanced over and asked if I was feeling okay. I smiled, but my eyes began to tear up because the reality had hit me. "I will never put him into his crib again. Ever. Last night was the last time Braeden will ever sleep in his crib." That part of raising this child was done, and I wasn't ready for it. Time really did pass quickly.

I saw in that one moment all the endings and new beginnings that this child—and my children to come—had in store for me, making every moment we shared even more precious, as impossible as that was.

Shane was born on a mild spring day at the end of March. Sam had grown absolutely enormous toward the end, so much so that people often asked if she was carrying multiples—she was huge! She looked like a cartoon, with a gigantic belly on her slim frame. I was not the only one to suggest that she get induced to deliver early because she was in such discomfort, but her doctor refused to consider it. "You're running a much higher risk of C-section if you induce early. Wait until you are past full-term, and then we can discuss it."

Sam began labor on the morning of March 30, the baby's due date. After a full day of contractions, when her spasms were close enough together we checked into the hospital and things progressed from there.

They set her up with a Pitocin drip. Sam was now in excruciating pain, which was very tough to witness. She finally gave in and agreed to some pain meds, after which things were less stressful—until the baby moved inside her. I swear this baby shifted over to the side, like it might want to come out that way instead. The nurse saw it too, and she flashed me a fake smile, saying, "I'm just going to go get the doctor now."

Our doctor walked in, took a moment to analyze the situation, and then said, calmly, "Sam, you are dilating just fine, but now you are swelling closed again. I think we may need to C-section you to get this baby out."

They prepped her for the C-section as I anxiously dressed in my scrubs and nifty cap. Now I really didn't know what to expect, but I knew it was going to freak me out a bit. All I could think of was the *Alien* movie and God knew what was waiting for us in that delivery room with Sam's massive belly. I held her hand as they made the incision. I knew right there and then why being a doctor was definitely out of the question for me. But as terrifying as this whole procedure was, I could not take my eyes off her stomach, watching the whole thing unfold. From his head to the rest of his body, they pulled out the largest baby any of us had ever seen.

"Oh my goodness! Look at the size of this baby!" someone said.

They held the baby for Sam to see and then took him over to the heat lamps to clean him up. Sam looked over at him. "He looks fine to me," she said. Remember, she'd been given all those pain meds.

I just started to cry again because I'm a fricking baby myself. But I had to admit, this was one big, beautiful baby!

The staff quickly organized a pool to guess his weight. I followed the nurse out with Shane Haaken to watch him being cleaned and weighed, camera in hand to mark this moment in history. His body was literally off the scale—his head hanging over on one side and his feet flopping off the other. We went back to the operating/delivery room and she made the announcement: "Twelve pounds, six ounces!"

Nobody won the bet on his weight—nobody had guessed over twelve pounds, anyway.

Overcome with elation and amazement, I leaned in to my lovely, amazing wife and whispered in her ear. "Twelve pounds, six ounces, Sam . . . it's the *twins*." And we shared a poignant, joyful cry together.

A LEGENDARY JOURNEY

SOMETIMES, THINGS HAPPEN just the way they are supposed to.

In the end, we got our little girl. Octavia Flynn was born on October 16, 2005, at a mere eight pounds, eight ounces. Upon seeing her for the first time Sam said, "She looks so tiny!" (After Shane, any baby would.)

Little Tavia completes my incarnation as a father. Little boys are a dad's dream, but this little girl is even more—she is everything. She is as girly as possible, and she evokes the most protective, paternal instincts in me. She dotes on me as only a little angel can, with butterfly kisses, coy grins, and the most beguiling snuggles. And every night at bedtime when she was in the crib, we sang songs and laughed until the sandman came to visit and she had no choice but to fall asleep.

Because they change so quickly and dramatically, my kids have brought to me an unlikely peace. Life, as we all must come to accept, is transient. The illness took so much from me in an instant, and with each passing day, now, my babies are gone too. My toddler Braeden has disappeared like a wave on the sand. I can no longer easily swing him around by his feet, much to our mutual dismay. But in his place there exists a nine-year-old with remarkable qualities and talents that the two-year-old version never even suggested. Every day my kids show me I cannot dwell in the past if I am to appreciate the gift that is the present.

I am more forgiving these days. I started with myself.

I practice patience.

I have learned to let things go, to reject frustration and anger as the extra baggage they are. No one is really strong enough to carry that weight and live to tell of it. I spent a good deal of energy directing anger at people and circumstances that were impervious (as they always are). That wasted effort hurt me far more than it ever touched them. My single-minded focus on my career, my extreme drive to produce, my devotion to a TV character that I let define me—all culminated in a cataclysmic shift, a literal and figurative loss of balance.

Now, as a father, a husband, and a guy who loves his work, my scales are steady.

God tapped me on the shoulder, with an aneurysm that might have been a small thing. It wasn't. It was an enormous, life-changing, fortunate event that continues to affect me, and it will for the rest of my life.

My strange brush with death, along with the battle for health that ensued, abruptly and profoundly transformed my world. In time a quiet strength gradually returned, my symptoms slowly abated, my tolerance grew, and I became not simply renewed but actually reinvented. In spite of myself, I eventually began to see beyond the losses and appreciate the rewards of this changed life. The act of suffering does not make you a victim—only your point of view can do that. Even loss can enrich.

And in giving you receive. Before getting sick I had begun to focus on educating children in creating healthy lifestyles and productive lives. A World Fit For Kids!, my after-school mentoring program, has grown to serve twelve thousand young people each year. Its positive effects shining back on me during my recovery gave me another kind of hope, one outside of myself.

Insights were hard won, coming only after years of struggle and disappointment as well as an endless battle of wills between the part of me that wanted happiness and peace and the part that ceaselessly pointed out my failures and frustrations. My personality and situation consigned me to endure alone, but I was sentenced to solitary anyway because I didn't believe anyone could ever truly know my challenges unless it actually happened to them. I was only partly justified. Aneurysm is a word most people don't understand. Stroke, too.

Aneurysms are so varied in their effects they almost demand modifiers (cerebral or aortic, for instance). Risk factors for getting an aneurysm include obesity, high blood pressure, smoking, or high alcohol consumption, yet I did not fit any of these descriptives. Most brain aneurysms go undetected until they rupture, causing severe brain damage or even death.

A stroke is defined as a restriction of the blood flow to any part of the brain, either due to a blood clot or burst blood vessel. According to the National Stroke Association, stroke is the leading cause of serious, long-term disability in the United States and the third most common cause of death. StrokeRecovery.com reports that strokes account for 10 percent of deaths in the United States every year. Close to 795,000 are diagnosed each year, and there are 6.5 million stroke sufferers in the United States alone.

Brain injury is an umbrella term that covers myriad issues. Under this banner stroke and concussion and brain aneurysm are brothers, equally disobedient and unwilling to be governed by any rules. I have huge empathy when the television announcer says a football player suffered a "mild concussion." Head injury is seldom mild if for no other reason than because it is lasting. It can be unrelenting and insidious. His concussion could well be something that player will be dealing with throughout the years to come.

As a thirty-eight-year-old with three strokes, I was a complete anomaly in a sea of inconsistency. Undeterred, the doctors first allotted me three months of healing time—an educated guess, but ultimately an arbitrary one. It saddens me today when I think of the incorrect medical predictions not only for me but also for others who may be similarly suffering. Modern medicine has a great many answers, and it certainly saved my life, but the power to heal is also the power to harm. A doctor can so easily and unwittingly take hope from a patient, and hope has enormous healing power. For a long time hope and faith were all I had. That is one reason I am making my story public now, to attest that there is always hope.

The fact remains that strokes and brain injuries are like snowflakes: entirely unique. The brain is an enigma, a riddle we have yet to solve, and therefore the ways in which it heals frequently seem without specific rules, making brain trauma often unbearably challenging. That said, all health struggles have similarities, and I hope that my story can be an inspiration to others to keep fighting and keep believing in possibilities, not statistics. After all, we are not in charge, and your perspective dictates your reality.

These days the physicality of *Hercules* is taking its toll in diverse ways. Three knee surgeries later, with another knee and a shoulder surgery scheduled, my body is succumbing to the years I demanded too much of it. All the fights and injuries I sustained are clamoring to be remembered now. The endless days of lifting weights, even before *Hercules*, mixed in with my football, basketball, baseball, and jogging, are catching up to me, though I have no regrets about them.

My health crisis and its long-term effects are also simply part of my life now. I still suffer from mild panic and anxiety. My sensitivity to medications renders them all but useless, though I have gained an understanding of my brain's chemical sensitivities and how those can drive my emotions. I still suffer migraines, but they seldom lay me out for an hour, much less days at a time. I often have residual arm pain from the circulation loss and nerve damage, but you'd never know it to look at me, much like the rest of my symptoms. And although I still have a blind spot in about 10 percent of my vision, my brain has adjusted quite well.

What's more, my sight is better today than ever before. The knowledge that I gained through this painful journey has made me a better, stronger man today. Among other things, my health crisis taught me the great lesson that *resting* is also a doing—and a necessity. I found usefulness for it that I never recognized before having children. Now, early in the morning, when I am working in my office and one of my children comes in for a morning cuddle, I stop everything. It is a favored moment for me, adjourning to my couch to hold my child quietly, feeling his or her small, trusting weight upon me. I say that grateful prayer again. Sam has said that I was moving so fast before the strokes that I would have missed this type of moment. Perhaps she's right.

Sam is an incredible partner on my journey, someone upon whom I easily depend. She is my link, my resource, and my advocate. Happily, we've weathered "for worse" and hope to appreciate "for better" until . . . well, you get the rest of it. She understands I am a work in progress. My appreciation of her runs deeper than any physical issues can touch.

Our beloved days of diapers and soothers, car seats and cribs are gone now. The babies have disappeared, but in their place I have three beautiful, boisterous, quick-witted children.

We drive to the beach (yes, I drive now again—another thing to be grateful for). Braeden, in the passenger seat next to me, says, "Daddy, what makes this sound? BTHFSSSTHSSTHSHCK!"

"I haven't a clue. What makes that sound?" I answer, laughing.

"I do," he says simply, with a proud, mischievous smile. "Didn't you just hear me?"

He loves to make people laugh, and his siblings and I gladly oblige him.

Shane asks me to turn on the radio. Our song, Journey's "Don't Stop Believing" comes on, and the kids immediately start shrieking. It is one of the few songs they have all claimed as their own. It is a great song from my college days, by one of my favorite groups. And my three small miracles know all the words.

CPSIA information can be obtained at www.ICGtesting.com
Printed in the USA
LVOW08s0748100914

403251LV00001B/1/P